THE ROLLER COASTER OF EMOTION
IN COUPLES THERAPY

Susan Thau PhD, PsyD
Sondra Goldstein PhD

S & S Publishing | Los Angeles, CA

© 2022 Susan Thau and Sondra Goldstein

All rights reserved. No part of this publication may be reproduced, stored in a retrieval system, or transmitted in any form or by any means electronic, mechanical, photocopying, recording or otherwise, without the prior written permission of the publisher.

Published by
S & S Publishing | Los Angeles, CA

> Publisher's Cataloging-in-Publication Data
> Thau, Susan.
>
> The roller coaster of emotion : in couples therapy /
> Susan Thau, PhD, Psy.D, and Sondra Goldstein, PhD. –
> Los Angeles, CA : S & S Pub., 2022.
>
> p. ; cm.
>
> ISBN13: 978-0-9601125-0-0
>
> 1. Couples therapy. 2. Marital psychotherapy. I. Title.
> II. Goldstein, Sondra.
>
> RC488.5.T43 2022
> 616.89156—dc23

Project coordination by Jenkins Group, Inc. | www.jenkinsgroupinc.com

Front cover design by T. Dwayne Johnson
Interior design by Brooke Camfield

Printed in the United States of America
26 25 24 23 22 • 5 4 3 2 1

Contents

	Introduction	v
	A Primer on How to Read This Book	xi
Chapter 1	Couples Therapy Begins	1
Chapter 2	Attachment in Couples	25
Chapter 3	Moving in the Right Direction	31
Chapter 4	Bring on the Addiction	45
Chapter 5	Hopelessness	57
Chapter 6	The Body and Brain in Couples	65
Chapter 7	Slow Down and Listen	75
Chapter 8	Implicit to Explicit	83
Chapter 9	Couples and Patterns	103
Chapter 10	Zoom and Everything Changes	111
Chapter 11	The Path Taken	139
Chapter 12	In Conclusion	165
	Questions for the Reader	169
	References	173
	About the Authors	177
	Acknowledgments	179

Introduction

Couples therapy is a mystery to most people. During difficult times in marriage, partners wonder, "Should we go to couples therapy to solve these problems?" or "Can we make our relationship better?" In the United States today, about 129 million people are married or cohabitate and millions more are in an exclusive dating relationship as a couple. While the difficulties affecting a specific couple are a personal matter, whether a couple remains stable and functioning affects not only the couple but also society as a whole. In some ways we all pay the price when a couple becomes unstable. But more about this later.

Who are we and why we are writing this book?

We are clinical psychologists who have worked for many years with a broad spectrum of couples, from those who have worries about a difference in perspective to others who are moving toward the edge of the partnership cliff. We have both been in long-term marriages, raised children, and established our own careers.

About twenty-five years ago, we met in a study group where we became focused on understanding the relationship between our brains, emotions, and relational dynamics. After studying and working together, we became collaborators due to our shared interest. We began to lecture and write because these matters were obviously significant in clinical work, and we hoped to educate our colleagues in relational dynamics. We were drawn to couples work, because it allowed us to use and consider the relational concepts and our knowledge about emotions.

We have seen over and over the improvements in relationships that can occur when partners become attuned to what goes on between them, when they stop the blame game. However, it is not only the partners that are changed. This process affects and changes us as therapists. This may seem strange, but we do feel more expansive and engaged in life from working with these couples. Because this work has been so life-enhancing, we decided that we wanted to de-mystify the elements of being in a partnership. We hope you'll feel curious about learning what goes on during the process and what can interrupt the good feelings and connection that are present when the relationship begins. We hope our book will help readers be less anxious about the unknown aspect of being in a partnership, and in some cases, it might help some to consider seeking professional help.

Why does this topic matter so much and have such far-reaching impact? Our intent has been to help couples understand how and why their relationship is not functioning well, and help them learn how to put their relationship on a better footing. We are passionately committed to helping others know that they can change their lives and their brains—even if they have had difficulty and disadvantages while in their families of origin. We are committed to the belief that couples can learn how to have a secure experience even in the face of so much suffering in all walks of life. This skill is particularly important at this time.

We began this project in the midst of the COVID pandemic. The health crisis and its need for sheltering in place quickly caused an increase in family and relational strain. This made sense to us because the response to this pandemic changed everything about the way we worked and how we lived. Some individuals were able to adapt and cope with the changes that occurred, while others—especially those who struggle with change, and whose rigidity predated the pandemic—suffered greatly. In partnerships, when one person begins to flail, the other is often drawn into the vortex of this pain. A partner's emotional stability (or lack of) is transferred to those who are attached to this person.

Inspiration comes in various ways. The seeds of this book began while meeting in case consultation, a practice that occurs even when the therapist has been working in the field for a long time. A colleague, Donn Peters, talked about how he had wanted to write a book about our practice as therapists, not for clinicians, but for people who know little about couples therapy. Donn inspired us with his interest in David Brooks' book *The Social Animal*, in which Brooks tells the story of a fictional couple and how they healed their relationship. Brooks challenges the typical notions of "success" as he traces the unfolding lives of Harold and Erica from their families of origin to their marriage and beyond. Along the way, he addresses a revolution in thought proposing that the unconscious mind is far more important than the conscious one. Brooks states, "I want to show you what this unconscious mind looks like when it is flourishing, when the affections and aversions that guide us every day have been properly nurtured, the emotions properly educated" (2011, xii). While the idea that our affections, aversions, and emotions need to be nurtured and educated may come as a surprise to most readers, nonetheless, it is true.

Our book is a story that includes commentary and explanation. It is a story of a fictional couple, John and Maria and their marriage—how it began, how it proceeded through the various stages of life, and how they eventually find themselves in trouble, and seeking marital therapy. Relating back to David Brooks' proposition, John and Maria, stumbled in the challenges of their relationship because they began cycling up and down, as if on a roller coaster, when they attempted to understand and be with each other emotionally. In the chapters that follow, we offer a narrative of our fictional couple in imagined therapy sessions that have been pulled from our years of experience doing couples therapy. These narratives are not representative of any one couple, but are a compilation and confabulation of many partnerships. Some of the stories are borrowed from our own marriages.

We intersperse the narrative chapters with several chapters on theory. We use theory to help clarify and explore the process in the previous chapter, and invite the reader to appreciate the myriad interactions involved. How we use theory—informed by our own experiences, intuitions, and understandings—to assist the couple before us is part science and part art.

In the sessions, we put forth a narrative from our couple and include some of the therapist's own insights. *These inside thoughts are identified separately by a thinking-head icon and the thoughts themselves in italics.* If it is true that we all live with a complex set of interwoven, interdependent relationships, then the therapist's experiences are also of value. We include some of our own process—which has been highly edited for obvious reasons—to further pull back the curtain and illuminate the reciprocal dynamics in action. Our goal is to enhance your knowledge and understanding of human relationships—yours especially, as well as others.

Understanding, however, is not enough. We hope to motivate you to become aware of your feelings, to make changes in those areas of life that interfere with a sense of balance, to deal with discomforts that are experienced, and to encourage self-reflection as a means of stabilizing and helping personal growth. The reader may discover parts of himself/herself in John and Maria's story, not because of being exactly the same, but because witnessing the struggle will likely encourage introspection and a consideration about living one's own life. We look forward to being a guide on this exciting and revealing inner journey.

Sondra Goldstein and Susan Thau

A Primer on How to Read This Book

This book is written to help you understand what goes on in couples therapy, and what goes on internally in each participant—the therapist and the two partners. Each participant is engaged and reacts to whomever they are speaking with as well as the observer. We have attempted to deal with what you would see externally, but that is just the beginning.

We have also tried to depict what goes on with the therapist as she engages—at times easily and at times with great difficulty—with each participant. The complexity of these interactions cannot be overstated. The person directly involved with the therapist is being evoked, but so is the other partner who is an observer. This is crucial in terms of the complicated feeling states that these interactions involve. This is another aspect of the roller-coaster ride.

In order to clarify these processes dynamically, we have written about the therapist's inside thoughts. These thoughts are always set aside as they may not relate to the actual external situation. When they are written into the narrative, they are identified by a thinking-head icon with the content in *italics*.

Another feature of this book is the theory and explanations that are interspersed throughout the story. Our intention is to provide a way for you to pursue aspects of the therapeutic process in a more in-depth way, should you choose to do so. These theory and process notations are identified with a text-box symbol.

Our general focus is the couple, the therapist, the theory and clinical process. We want you to learn about John and Maria and their mutual struggle to feel connected and safe with each other. You will get to know the therapist as a very real person with her own feelings and challenges that emerge from her life experiences and through her work with John and Maria. Knowing who the therapist is and how this impacts the partners individually may be surprising at times. The clinical theory and process are laid out as something that can be further studied as part of this work.

We hope that as you become involved in reading this book, these three aspects will become even more interesting to you personally and enhance your own journey as you reflect on what these characters and their encounters awaken in you. Why are you drawn to one of these characters or not? Why does a particular subject feel important or cause you to feel annoyed or even angry? Why do you remember a particular exchange and what is it triggering in you? We hope the beam of light that we are shining will beckon you to go deeper into your own inner world.

Chapter 1

Couples Therapy Begins

Do you ever wonder what is happening behind the closed door of a therapist's office? Perhaps you are curious about who is in there and what they're talking about. Maybe you have wondered if you know them—especially if someone you are close to is actually seeing a therapist. Or you may have toyed with the idea of walking in there to get the therapist's take on that nagging problem you've been having with your own partner. This book takes you behind that closed door. Together, we will observe and examine the experience of a couple in the process of going to therapy.

Don't worry that you're being voyeuristic. The couple is fictional, constructed out of our experiences with different couples seen over the years. What is not fictional, however, is our exploration of ourselves as therapists. Because of our earnest commitment to widening the appreciation of the therapeutic process, we hope to expand your understanding and grasp of the value and possibilities of being in therapy. We want to replace any misconceptions and fears you may have with a deepening appreciation of our human complexities, and a respect for the effort required to create order and meaning of often-disabling confusions of life.

It's normal to be curious about the persona of the therapist. What type of person sits with others and actively listens to their pain and worries? How can you tell this person—someone you've never known—the deepest, darkest pains of your life? Has this therapist ever grappled with the problems plaguing you? How can the therapist possibly know what you are going through? It comes down to this, "How can—or will—I ever totally trust this person?" We will address these and a myriad of other issues as we go through John and Maria's therapeutic experience. Consider there is a door that separates the clinical space from the outside world, but you are being invited to sit alongside during the sessions. Let me give you an idea of what you can expect.

In this first session you will meet John and Maria and immediately see how they begin to trigger each other. This dynamic is called their dance because the particular pattern of disengaging usually follows certain specific steps. You will see how the therapist—the observer—puts together a picture of this process for the couple so they can begin to make sense of their own moves in this dance. Notice how unprocessed pain and wounds begin to manifest and how these have to be brought into the healing process. This is illustrated in the dynamic between Maria and the therapist. You will be learning about this phenomenon, called transference, in this chapter and throughout the book. It is important for you to know about transference because it happens to all of us as feeling, emoting human beings.

Let's jump in and meet John and Maria and learn more about what brought them to seek out a therapist.

John and Maria's First Session

When I listened to my voicemails one morning, I heard an unfamiliar and tentative voice. Maria introduced herself and told me that she and her newly married husband were already having "big problems." She said that they had been referred by a friend and asked me to return her call.

This matter of getting a new referral is an interesting and at times a challenging situation. Probably most of us in the field of mental health are sensitive to hearing and responding to the pain and distress of others. If someone is seeking help, is asking to be seen, already there is the built-in conundrum, the risk involved in being vulnerable with a total stranger. I was glad to hear someone had referred Maria since I am more receptive to making space for new clients when I know the referring person in some way. I do feel the sense of a slight risk about opening my office—or, really, my heart—to someone when I don't know anything about them.

When I returned Maria's call, I learned that she was from Italy, and had married John after an intensely romantic international courtship. Just hearing about that caused me to pause, to see a "red flag," which is what I call my intuition about a potential problem. I mused about how they could know each other if they had mostly been playing together in vacation mode.

This phone contact is real enough. Imagine the importance a brief phone call carries in determining whether you want to work with a person. Are you able to talk with someone briefly on a phone call and feel comfortable inviting them in, to even consider becoming extensively involved with them? Each therapist has his or her own way of handling this first contact, but in a strange way it feels like being on a speed date. I listen carefully, ask a few specific questions, and then feel my way around involving myself further with them. Initial contact through email is even more limited and possibly problematic when it comes to making this decision.

In that first return phone call, Maria told me that she and John were constantly fighting, she was having problems at work, and she was wondering if she should go back to Italy. "Why should I stay here if I have nothing, only a bad relationship and possibly no job?" I found myself already thinking, *This is going to be one hard case*. But her aloneness tugged at my heart, and I found myself wanting to help her. Because of my feelings evoked in listening to her distress, I scheduled an appointment for John and Maria the next week.

As I opened the waiting room door for our first in-person appointment, it was apparent that something had gone awry between them that was still in play. Not even knowing these people, I felt myself bracing for what they were bringing into my office. The tension hung in the air like a thick fog.

John and Maria did not walk together, and their body language conveyed an uncomfortable, angry energy. Although I was distracted by the negative energy, I also noticed that there were racial differences. John's swarthy, dark complexion was in marked contrast to Maria's pale coloring. I made a mental note that we would have to take this up and understand how it affects their partnership.

Before I even extended a welcome, Maria blurted out, "This is just impossible. I live with a man who is mostly not present. I can tell him over and over what I need, and it's like he just doesn't really hear it. It feels like he lives in his own world. He comes into reality, and a life with me, only when he chooses to."

She gave me an example of how dismissive he could be. It was not a major event, but it had just happened that past weekend when they were visiting with a relative, and so it was fresh in her mind. She thought it would give me a better idea about why she gets so upset. Maria told John that she needed to be home to participate in a call at a certain time. She thought she made her needs clear so that both things—visiting at the family gathering and the phone call—could take place smoothly. In curt words, Maria explained that she signaled John on a number of occasions, but each time he continued to talk and further engage with the others rather than her.

And then, still in an angry voice, she added, "But what made it worse, really upsetting, was what happened when I tried to explain how this was affecting me. I was really trying to be calm, but I couldn't believe that he was just ignoring me as if I had never said anything about the phone call I needed to make. It made me feel crazy, perfectly crazy. I do know that the way I handled it made him go on the offensive and tune me out even more. I wish he would understand that when he doesn't talk to me, it makes me even more upset, and I feel like I don't matter to him at all."

She explained that she tried to tell him how upset and disappointed she felt. Glaring at him, she said, "He just stared at me, with such cold eyes, and I could tell that he was sending me a message that he's done with me." Then her voice became a bit softer and she added, "It's always been that way. It's never going to change."

The Roller Coaster of Emotion

Dr. S: So you feel that you're ignored by John, and that he really doesn't notice the pain you're in?

Maria: He never notices the pain I'm in. The minute I try to tell him my feelings, about anything at all, he gets all quiet and then he stops looking at me. It is impossible, just impossible, to be with someone who just goes away. All this means to me is that he doesn't care at all.

Dr. S: John, how is this for you? Please tell me what's going on inside you when you hear Maria protesting about how alone and uncared for she feels.

John: I can see her boiling, and so irritated, which makes me feel kind of crazy. I can't even figure out what she's upset about and then she yells at me for seemingly nothing. I was just talking to our family and suddenly she seemed to lose it. I feel like she's mad at me all the time and it never makes any sense.

> **THERAPIST INSIDE THOUGHTS:** *This is a typical withdrawer feeling. "I don't get why you're so mad at me." Withdrawers feel unjustly accused, and they often express an internal confusion. They quickly feel criticized and are easily shamed. I'll need to take it slow with this man to really get behind the wall of shame and defense.*

Maria *interrupts:* There you go again—blaming me, making me the bad person, saying that I lose it, and that it is all my fault. It's not just me John, it's you too. You never seem to realize what you've done and how that affects me. And you're doing it right here, right now. I am so glad that this therapist gets to see how quickly you blame me!

> *Oh, what have I gotten myself into? Are they going to be one of those highly escalated couples? Can I calm them down, especially with the stakes being so high? She said that she was thinking of going back to Italy and to her family. This feels like so much responsibility. I've got to take this slowly and be able to hold a space without getting afraid myself. All right, I say to myself, breathe slowly; you know what to do. First, slow her down so she can begin to engage in the process. But that's tricky because she may get even more reactive, and then I'll become the bad guy.*

Dr. S: Maria, I know you have a lot to say. I can see how upset you are, and that you're concerned that I won't see what this is like for you. Please give me a moment to talk with John, and then I'll come back to you, I promise.

Dr. S: John, it sounds as though you feel like you're getting attacked all the time and that it doesn't make sense to you because you feel like you've done what you can, you're a good guy, and that it is never enough. So what happens, John, when you feel this way? What's it like inside for you, in your body?

John: It's like my insides are turning upside down, and when I can't stop them, I start to feel like I am a nut case. I just want to get away from her and stop this whole thing. I can't think of anything when this happens.

The Roller Coaster of Emotion

Dr. S: You mean it kind of takes over your mind so that you feel like you're tumbling in space, you're nowhere.

> *My goal is trying to tune into his profound aloneness and state of mind. He is confused when it comes to understanding Maria's feelings of disappointment and hopelessness about their relationship. He can't seem to make sense of Maria's feelings. It's like he is saying, "I've been a good guy, why are you angry with me?"*

John: Tumbling in space is too small. I feel like I'm losing my grip because I can see her, but she's beyond my reach, and I don't really want to be near her anyway because she's like a firecracker that's exploding.

> *I am watching them escalate, especially Maria. As John is talking, her face is becoming more and more contorted. I'm feeling a bit trapped with these very intense people, especially after my morning. But I can also feel Maria's pain, which she expresses like an angry cat that is howling and hissing. And I am also concerned that John is slipping away. Why wouldn't he? He's scared, too, because he is not able to engage with Maria when her anger is so palpable and hot. But what can I do? They are both off and running away from each other. High-arousal amygdala hijack, that what this is. I will have to explain this to them later when the tsunami is over. I know that I have to get them interested in what they are doing, what actions they are taking that actually push them further and further away from each other. Right now, their automatic responses—their defenses—are*

causing more reactivity in their moves with each other. When there have been too many experiences of feeling uncared for, attachment becomes fragile.

I am seeing their attachment dance where each partner is coping in a way that makes sense given what they have felt about themselves and others. In the core of her being, Maria feels that she is not worthy of being listened to unless she subjugates herself to John. In this session, she is already exhibiting concerns that I may be more sensitive to John, and not really interested in how she feels or what goes on in her heart. So given these deeply held feelings, she rages at him to signal the miserable state she is in. It is as if the more he withdraws and dims, the more she lights up in an attempt to urgently send her major signal of distress. This is all they know how to do, and I have to create enough safety in this room to allow them to get in touch with what is going on inside, particularly their unprocessed pain and feelings. What I know within these first few minutes is that she feels unnourished and alone. When it comes to partnering, that is definitely a lethal combination.

Dr. S: Maria, I can see that you are having a hard time here. Every word John speaks seems to make you more distressed. Can you tell me more about this feeling that you're having?

Maria: You bet I'm distressed. He doesn't pay any attention to me, and now he's complaining that my distress is making him get upset inside. What's the point? His words tell me that he doesn't care anymore, that I don't matter to him at all. That's what it comes down to. I just know I have no place here or with him.

The Roller Coaster of Emotion

I am learning about Maria even though I do not know much about her earlier experiences. I sense that she is used to being with others who were unable to recognize her suffering. It's as if the minute she feels the other's pain, she feels there is no place for hers. In this instance, when John expresses that he is upset or has suffered, she feels blamed for her feelings and becomes both angry and reactive. John feels inadequate about his ability to communicate in any way, and once he feels her anger, it signals to him that he has failed. That is the dance that painfully takes them each to separate corners.

Maria is trying to get John's attention, and signal him about her acute distress. Her core basic feeling is that she is miserably alone and uncared for. So, based on this felt experience, she has started to pull away in anger and rage. Her brain is signaling her that she's in danger and so—predictably—she is in flight. I need to help this couple understand what they are fighting against, but I also need to keep Maria present because she is starting to go into a rage state. John is revealing his fragile sense of self regarding feeling emotional incompetency. Of course, this didn't begin with Maria but now it's being played out over and over again. This guy feels inadequate about his ability to communicate in any way, and once he feels her anger, it signals him that he's failed. They are both in a constant state of scaring each other even further and further away.

Dr. S: Oh, Maria, it must seem so impossible, doesn't it, when you just want John to talk to you. But either he isn't there or he seems intent on getting at you with his comments on your anger, which I'm sure feels so unjust.

> *I keep wondering what has happened to Maria that she is in such a rage. I don't know about her life yet, but I am sure there is a reason why John's behavior triggered her. One thing she mentioned was about working so hard all the time. I can relate to that. I know that is a dark place I can go to when I feel that all I do is work, and that it is taken for granted. It is not a good feeling for sure. Watching and feeling Maria's anger and rage, I felt my own shame as I wondered if I look like her when I am angry. I want to get away from her, and even have a searing thought that maybe my husband wants to withdraw from me. I had better stop myself from going there right now. But it is awakening some empathy for her when a moment ago I had none. I have to help her, to stay with her—even her angry self—because I truly know how painfully lonely that kind of unprocessed pain can be.*

Maria: You're right, it feels impossible and now I'm watching you and feeling that you're looking at me and judging me as well. Everyone thinks that I'm too intense and too demanding. You probably do, too.

The Roller Coaster of Emotion

> *I need to help John and Maria. What do I do with Maria's feelings that I am judging her for getting so upset and emotional? I know I can't just tell her to stop feeling that way. She is broadcasting loud and clear that she does not feel safe, so I need to let her know that this concerns me and that I will listen to her experience as well as what is happening to her. Her reaction tells me about past experiences that she has had with others. This is probably what happens to her when she feels unsafe or has feelings about this kind of situation. And if there is no safety, who wouldn't have those feelings? Will I be able to let her know that I understand how important her feelings are, that her anger makes sense when she feels threatened? I want to talk to her about building walls, but I am not sure that she will be open with me when I—in her eyes—have become just another judge.*

Dr. S: Maria, I am feeling your walls go up to protect yourself from any more hurt. I am hearing that you think that I'm a part of the problem and that maybe I'm judging you as well. I hope you'll let me know what has happened so that we can look at it together. Can you help me with this?

Maria: Well, if you really want to know, I saw your face when I was raging at John and I just know that you're like the others who are always critical of me and blame me for my emotions.

Dr. S: Oh, Maria, I get that you saw me wince, but it's not because you were so angry. I can see why you thought that, and I'd like to share something personal if that is all right. (She nods and looks at me a bit skeptically.) I am a human just like you, and your reaction reminded me of my own struggles when I feel that I am trying to get my feelings out, when I am feeling misunderstood. There is nothing like that searing, painful moment which feels so big and complete. You are looking at John and he feels like he's the enemy who does not care at all. Am I getting that right? That's a human reaction when you feel alone and uncared for. It's like you're saying, "See me, I am drowning in the feeling that you're not even there."

Maria: Are you saying that you have gotten so angry that even you have felt like you want to get away from the person you're with? I have always felt like there's something wrong with me. Are you saying that this is a regular human response? I just can't believe that others, even you, have felt this way.

> *First of all, I am glad I could do this because I feel I am creating safety in this process, and now hopefully I can help these two very scared people turn to each other. But I am uncomfortable that she knows about my anger when we barely know each other. She is asking me about being human, about feelings, about being normal. What does she think of me now that I have let it out that I can be really angry at times? She is trying to figure out what is human and what is normal. She is essentially trying to make sense of her behavior, which is what we do as humans. I know I need to be real with her or she will see right through me. This is hard because it's challenging to expose myself and my own vulnerabilities.*

Dr. S: Maria, I can hear you struggle with what you feel. It sounds like you are trying to figure out the depth of your anger, and if you are different from others because at times you feel so emotional. We need to connect with what has happened that has caused this reaction, but all of us as humans—myself included—feel anger at times. It happens quickly and without thought; it's a feeling that just comes on when we feel uncared for by the individual who is supposed to be our person, supposed to be there when we need support and caring. When this happens, it is like our partner feels like an enemy because—in that moment—the heart connection feels as if it has evaporated, disappeared.

Maria: Well, that is how I feel sometimes. And all I can think about is that I want John to know just how much I am suffering. I want him to get it, and feel bad for the way he is treating me.

Dr. S: It's like you turn up the volume so he'll know exactly how you're feeling, but instead of coming toward you, all you want to do, John, is get away, as far away as possible. Sadly, this further escalates Maria's feelings that you just don't care. Both of you start to feel that awful sense of loneliness, and everything that's ever kept you together seems to be gone. Neither of you can remember the connection between you when you're in one of these dark places. It's as if the world has become empty of all love and caring. That's what happens when we feel that the person that we are most connected to isn't there at all.

> *At this point, I can see that I could talk about the ways we process anger, how our amygdala gets triggered, the hidden meanings from the present situation, and even unconscious triggers. Maria's sense of being invisible was not only based on a specific event between her and John, but was also rooted in the myriad moments and events of her earlier life where she was either overlooked, felt unsatisfied, or had longings that were not met. John had failed to recognize this. When Maria confronted him about how dismissive his actions had felt, he felt unjustly attacked and criticized and became defensive, which left Maria feeling alone and uncared for.*

Upon reflection, this session could have gone another way. After I shared information about myself, Maria could have continued to be angry and turned it back on me. She could have held on to her reactive anger, as well as her feelings that I had tried to distract and minimize her anger, which was the opposite of what I was trying to do. If this had happened, that first session could have been our one and only because if one partner feels misunderstood, this derails the beginning process. To do couples therapy, both partners have to feel safe enough that they can sit with their feelings without a sense of judgment or interference from the therapist. Knowing this, I was particularly concerned when Maria felt judged by me so early in the process. When there is no previous foundation, the treatment is highly unlikely to go forward. Of course, I am extremely glad that she was able to hear my associations. This outcome gave me a clearer sense of what might be helpful in the future.

Introduction to John and Maria

Who are these people you just met? As humans, our behavior comes from our lived experience. My initial goal is to understand what happened in the lives of John and Maria, their earlier connections, what worked, what felt good, and what happened that was not heart- and connection-building. How these earlier connections evolved provides me with a deeper appreciation for why this relational distress is happening.

Maria and John presented outwardly as young, attractive, and educated. But while they share many things in common, there are major differences between them that include their culture, the worlds they came from, and their ethnicity. John is a biracial man, an American through and through. Maria was born and raised in Italy, in a coastal resort outside Napoli. I asked them to tell me the story of their relationship and about the family that they each came from.

Their romance began as a relational love story. John, in between jobs, feeling carefree and excited, was visiting Italy with some friends. One night in a café having a leisurely dinner, he heard conversation at the table nearby and laughter and gaiety that filled the room. He felt a sense of pleasure and interest. Who were those happy people? What was giving them such pleasure? He turned around and noticed the attractive woman at the end of the table who was telling a story and laughing with a lyrical quality. At that moment he thought, *I wish I knew her. She seems so interesting and filled with such energy.*

The evening progressed with both engaged in their own deep conversations with their friends. Time passed, and as the café closed and emptied, they were the only two tables left. John thought to himself that he wanted to meet the laughing woman. And then, as fate would have it, they were soon the only two people left in the room. John remembers that he went up to her, smiled, and said—in his rather imperfect Italian—that he enjoyed the sound of her laughter. As quickly as he spoke, she responded in English, "Thanks, I am glad that you appreciated that I was having a great evening."

After that first evening, their romance was somewhat of a whirlwind because John knew he would leave Italy in a few weeks.

Let's understand the differences that are factors in this partnership. John is biracial. What matters is how this is dealt with—or not—between the partners. We will get into that later, but let's learn about John's family and culture. John can trace his roots back to his paternal grandfather, a black man, who was born and raised in the South. John's paternal grandmother is Vietnamese. They met when John's grandfather was stationed in the Far East after WWII. Unlike many other relationships at the time, they stayed together and got married. John's father was born shortly after they came back to the States where his grandfather continued his career in the military.

John's father grew up in the 1950s, and faced a lot of challenges as a biracial man and an army brat living among other military families. He talked a lot about the challenges he faced as a biracial man in the South, who could never get a step ahead to stand up and move forward and felt passed over and kept out of advancement. What had given John's father more advantages was that as a good athlete, he had been recruited by the local college. There he met and married John's mother who was also from a military family. But the marriage took place because his mother became pregnant, and terminating the pregnancy was not an option. We can say that John's very conception occurred under stressful circumstances. His parents had neither planned nor wanted to have a child. John's mother identified herself as a Hispanic since her family came from Mexico. From the beginning, John's mother and father did not have a good foundation. John was an only child, just like his father had been, and his parents' relational problems were readily apparent to him even as a very young boy.

Later on, John's father explained that he found his wife's fragility attractive at first, but as time passed, he became irritated and bored with her and gradually pulled away. As a child, all John saw was conflict. When asked about his parents' relationship, he reported that he could not remember a time when they were not fighting. John claims that he did not really know what was happening, but he could hear the noise and his mother's seemingly endless bouts of crying. He hated this and wished it would stop, so—as a protective device—he would hum to himself and try to think of anything that would block out the sounds. In the mornings, no one would say anything to him, and they would each go about their days as if the arguments had never happened. John sometimes wondered if he imagined this but, of course, it kept happening so he eventually realized that it was real. He tried to tell himself that it didn't really matter because nothing would change. That was also not true, and so when his parents brought him into the living room one Sunday, he could tell from their faces that he was going to hear something bad.

His parents finally separated when he was about five and because of his age, John lived primarily with his mother. She had always struggled with anxiety, and the divorce left her in an even more precarious state. She became preoccupied with John and worried that he would be adversely affected by the split, but her hovering attention was difficult for him. He reported that—even early on—he wanted to "not have to deal with it. I felt her worries, and that made me want to get away." She was an anxious woman about most everything, and believed that if she didn't watch carefully, some danger might befall him.

At first his parents lived separately, which in some ways was all right. John preferred this because the fighting had stopped and he could go to sleep. But he continued to keep all of these concerns to himself. His mother went to live with her mother, and John did not like living with the two women. He felt that being around two sad, anxious women was more pressure than he could deal with.

His father remained in the same town for a while, but eventually moved to another state. By the time John was an adolescent, he went to live with his father because John and his mother were not getting along.

As a well-meaning military man, John's father promoted values that included being strong, effective, and doing what you have to do—no matter what you might feel. Emotions and feelings had no place in his father's world, but at least John no longer had to deal with his mother's anxious, intrusive behavior. Throughout these challenging years, the one place where John succeeded was school. Both parents put a high premium on education, and John was quite exceptional. His parents were extremely proud. John knew how to navigate through school, how to plan, study, and achieve. He was a born student, and scholastics came easily to him, but expressing feelings about himself or his experiences was not something he was able to do. He deduced what was expected of him and was above all vigilant about avoiding any conflict, large or small, that might overtake him. Conflict meant being in an emotional minefield and it was possible, even likely, that you would be destroyed. He would go along to get along, which seemed preferable to getting into an untenable emotional place. It was almost as if John's motto was, "I'll figure out what you want and need, and then I'll do it that way so that you'll be all right—maybe even happy—and leave me alone."

> *These details identify John's anxious/avoidant attachment style. While he is loved by his mother, he withdraws from her. Why? Because he believes that connecting to her would mean subjugating himself, and essentially, losing himself as a separate person. Keeping his emotional distance is his way of being safe and avoiding the pain of disappointing another person. This emotional state can be very destabilizing because of the constant movement between longing and fear.*

If you met John, it isn't that you would find him hard to get along with. In fact, his outwardly easygoing personality was very likeable. But it was hard to really know what John was feeling except when it came to sports teams and players that he cared about. He was also open about his concern for people—both private and public—who were treated unjustly or faced challenging situations. His overall kindness was apparent, but it was noteworthy that John rarely talked about himself, specifically his feelings or concerns. It was as if John and only John had a key to his private self, and he shared this territory with no one.

When he was in college, John looked easygoing because he seemed to accept just about anything that was going on. From the outside, his developmental journey seemed effortless. By societal standards, as he moved into young adulthood after college, he was quite accomplished. Externally, John was quite good looking. His dark coloring was distinguishing and he was obviously biracial. John's looks did not help him in the dating arena. He had brief relationships that never seemed to last.

How John felt about himself, or the situations and people he was with, remained pretty much a mystery, because he rarely talked about any of that. It was after one of these breakups with a former girlfriend that John traveled to Italy before he was scheduled to begin a new job.

* * *

Maria's life was very different than John's. She was the younger daughter in a traditional Italian family. Her mother was an anxious woman, heavily involved with caring for both her two daughters and her own parents. They lived with their extended family in the family complex. Life was comfortable enough, and there were few challenges until just before Maria's fourteenth birthday. In the middle of a holiday celebration, on the day before Easter, her life changed dramatically and permanently.

That morning, she woke to the sound of her mother screaming, only to learn that her father had had a massive heart attack and was dead. Her mother, who had not worked before, obviously had to keep going in spite of her intense grief. Maria and her sister lost their father, who had been the more easygoing of their two parents. In spite of this teenage trauma, Maria had an enduring sense of wanting more for herself than the very sheltered life that she came from.

Unlike her sister, Maria began to plan early for how she would leave her provincial life, go to New York, and become a successful person. She read American magazines, listened to American singers, and watched current television shows. She was a good student and mastered English easily so this dream was based on what she felt she could achieve. Her ambition was nurtured by several nuns who took her under their wing and encouraged her academic efforts and the excitement that followed. This contrasted to Maria's home life where her mother's grieving and despair did not abate.

Maria explained that she found dating relatively easy, and had had a series of boyfriends, although none of consequence. She also commented specifically on how John's dark skin tone had been an "attractor" for her that had sensual meaning in her eyes. She had a black boyfriend several years before she met John.

Maria took her studies seriously and created career goals, a direction that would allow her to be noticed by those around her. When she graduated from university, being fluent in English, she interviewed and was hired by an international marketing firm. This fluency in combination with her emotional ease helped her to advance in this company. And then she met John. He came into her life as if on cue when she was primed to make another career change. This was her chance to actually leave her past behind her and aim for a more positive future life.

By emigrating to America, and believing it would be the place where her life would finally begin, she wanted to move forward and not be tethered to the past, to her mother, or to the repressive patriarchal rules of the social structure she was raised in. This was her longed-for goal, even though it meant giving up the close family connections that had been her life.

This background of John and Maria's history is of considerable importance even though this is a story about their current relationship. We will be looking at how these earlier attachment experiences come in to play in their relational struggles today. This concept of attachment is an important part of who we are and how we function in our relationships.

Chapter 2

Attachment in Couples

We will continuously reference the word attachment throughout this book. In this chapter, we will take a look at attachment both as a theory and as a way to relate with others, how we connect. This book is all about connection, what makes it possible, and when it is not able to occur, what is interfering with this basic biological need.

Developed by John Bowlby (1979), attachment theory proposes that attachment patterns observed in infant-caregiver interactions play a vital role in human development "from the cradle to the grave" (1979, 129). Bowlby believed that children develop internal working models about relationships that are implicit, nonconscious guides for later adult attachment relationships. Bowlby hypothesized that these childhood attachment patterns could change later in life as a result of new emotional experiences and new mental representations of attachment relationships. Fortunately, internal working models may be altered and updated, allowing an "earned secure" attachment style as development continues. These ideas provide a hopeful framework for couples as more secure internal working models can be created through transformative interactions in the "safe base" of couples therapy.

Attachment theory provides a helpful framework for understanding adult couple relationships. Bowlby (1969, 1973) proposed that attachment bonds are characterized by: (1) proximity-seeking; (2) safe-haven behavior; (3) separation distress; and (4) secure-base behavior. All of these features of infant-caregiver bonds may be observed in couple relationships. The partners derive comfort and security from each other. Each partner wants to be with the other, particularly in times of stress. When one partner in a relationship threatens to be physically or emotionally unavailable, the other partner may protest.

Adult couple relationships parallel the attachment styles identified in infant-caregiver relationships. Hazan and Shaver (1987) presented groundbreaking research which showed that the three major childhood attachment styles (secure, insecure-avoidant, and insecure-ambivalent) are also found in adult romantic relationships. Hazan and Shaver (1994) proposed that attachment styles of couples can be viewed in terms of the answer to the question, "Can I count on this person to be there for me if I need them?"

If the answer is yes, in a positive and secure way, the partners feel confident that they may rely on each other, have open communication, and experience a flexible, cooperative relationship. If the answer is maybe, partners tend to have an insecure-ambivalent style, with vigilance about loss, and alternating clinging and angry demands for reassurance. If the answer is no, the partner's past history of abuse, neglect, or rejection may have left no hope for a secure relationship. In the resulting insecure-avoidant attachment style, the partner avoids closeness or dependency, denies the need for attachment, and views others with mistrust.

Attachment styles or schemas become implicit, nonconscious, procedural memory networks that are evoked in interpersonal experiences, and particularly in important attachment relationships. What this means is that we get triggered in our interactions with our partners because some unknown experience or issue is still active whether or not we can actually remember it. We carry these unthought, unknown memories which come into play when we are experiencing relational stress. Attachment schemas guide the selection of significant others and influence the emotions experienced within relationships. When a couple's attachment schema is challenged, or the attachment bond is breached, a couple may seek treatment. Knowledge of attachment styles and internal working models of relationships provides a perspective in couples therapy for understanding the underlying needs and longings in intimate relationships.

Couples therapy has traditionally been associated with developing communication skills as a means of building intimacy between partners. But frequently, this approach does not create lasting improvement. Couples may relapse into familiar patterns of conflict that become increasingly destructive. Integrating attachment theory into couples therapy places the emphasis on how couples can work together to help each other emotionally. Partners can learn how the linking of their nervous systems can at times create "emotional reverberations," and that these are an inevitable part of intense attachment to another person (Lewis et al., 2000, 131). When partners feel that they can turn to each other emotionally, which means feeling cared for even when they have their unique differences, the bond is deepened and the relationship becomes more secure.

Research involving the relational patterns between mothers and infants (Beebe and Lachmann, 2002) has shown that a baby needs the mother's watchful presence that observes and helps when the baby is in any form of distress. This finding is validated in couple dynamics, too. In couples treatment, the partners depend on the therapist to help them learn how to manage emotions together, an ability that may never have been learned, or if learned, has been eroded by unrepaired, continuing conflict. Recognizing the mutual and core need of being with another person, of giving and receiving care, legitimizes the basic need of benign caretaking, especially in stressful life conditions (Solomon, 1994). There is hope that by understanding each other better, by learning to read each other's verbal and nonverbal cues, and by gaining a deeper appreciation of their own level of arousal, the partners will become more adept at managing their emotions with each interaction, thereby strengthening their relationship. Fortunately, to be a "good enough" partner does not require 100 percent accuracy in empathy or availability but "just enough" to create safety in a couple relationship. Research has shown that an accuracy rating of 30 percent is enough to create a sense of safety in a couple relationship (Tronick, E.Z. & Gianino, A. 1986).

There is an ongoing struggle for the couple to answer the question, "Can I count on this person to be there for me?" The response provides insight into their attachment schemas. Couples therapy is about helping each partner understand his or her part in interrupting the attachment connection, both in overt and nonconscious ways. Each member of the couple must try to make sense of personal attachment needs, understand that perfect attunement is not the goal, and aim to repair the inevitable moments of disruption. Resilience and commitment are essential components of a truly loving and enduring relationship.

Secure attachments can be "earned" by intervention, most often in the form of therapy. Other secure relationships also help because as humans, we are deeply affected by those we are emotionally involved with. Because our brains are actually emotionally linked, a new attractor, the therapist, offers a fresh and more vitalizing perspective. The emotional center of our brain is in the limbic system and this process is known as limbic resonance. There are numerous models of treatment but what research shows is that a therapist's experience and ability to establish a good working relationship with a couple is what makes the difference. The primary aim for the couples therapist is to help establish a secure marital attachment necessary for healthy functioning.

John and Maria's Attachment Styles

We meet John and Maria as adults, but we can surmise about their attachment patterns from what we know about their history. It seems clear that John is an over-regulated person who avoids conflict and most types of emotional engagement if at all possible. He reported that he sought to avoid his mother's overbearing anxiousness, and in a sense, he spent his time trying to "keep away from" rather than being "engaged." This pattern of withdrawal and avoidance would have consequences later in life, of course, in his primary relationship.

Maria is quite the opposite, because she is intensely emotional, and at times even under-regulated. While she may have been pursuing

John for connection at first, Maria has been withdrawing and experiencing burnout because she felt that her needs for attachment were not being considered. From what she reports about her family of origin, she is likely ambivalently attached. She longs for emotional engagement, but looks for signs of misalignment and a lack of understanding. This type of reactivity complicates her primary relationship. We will be looking at these patterns as we proceed with their story.

Chapter 3

Moving in the Right Direction

John and Maria are back. I brace myself knowing that they are most likely going to start revving up, and I have to slow them down so that they can reflect on their relationship, make sense of the moves they are making, and recognize the messages of connection or disconnection they are communicating to each other. Frequently, individuals have never looked at the dynamics of their partnership and their contribution to keeping this disruptive cycle going.

Over the years I have often been asked, "Are you trying to save every relationship?" Working with couples, I have had to consider if I do hold that bias. What I know now is that I am a process consultant because I help people look at the way they relate to each other, and get interested in the messages they are transmitting. As creatures of habit, we don't often practice this self-reflection; instead, we repeat the same behaviors no matter how distressed we might feel. Keeping this in mind, let's look at Maria and John.

The Roller Coaster of Emotion

> *Maria and John sit down, again without really looking at each other. I am reading every movement and especially watching their faces for cues as to their state to prepare for what I am dealing with. I don't like to be taken by surprise, but I have to trust myself to be able to stay the course, even if they are quite upset. I plant my feet on the ground and feel the hardness beneath me. It is my personal way of stabilizing myself. I am sending my body a message to be calm, which helps with my own regulation. Here we go . . .*

Dr. S: Glad to see you again. In the last session we were just getting to know each other and you each explained why you've been so upset. Maria, you told me that you don't feel that you matter to John anymore because he seems so unconcerned with your needs and feelings. You talked about a situation where you felt thrown under the bus with him attending to everyone else but you. This situation confirmed your growing belief that there was no point in investing in this relationship. And you, John, expressed your sense that you cannot do anything right. You feel that even though you make an effort, it is never noticed. Because of this constant criticism of your behavior, you've begun to turn away from Maria because it is just too painful.

Maria: There is something I want to say. I've been thinking about all of this ever since we left your office. I just know that I shouldn't let him in, because if I let my guard down, I'm going to really be sorry. Why in the world would I want to trust him? I just knew that once he was no longer interested in me he'd be like everyone else in my life who left me, including my father—even though he didn't do it intentionally. When we first met, I tried to be there for him and of course now I feel foolish for expecting that same effort in return.

> *I am so concerned about the rigidity that I hear from Maria. Of course, it makes sense given her early experiences. She mentioned the loss of her father, so I'll have to get underneath that issue since this "unintended loss" definitely affected her. She's signaling that this is a raw spot that hurts and oozes like an open wound. I have to be careful not to push her too hard because she will just put her wall up. Using a protective wall of anger has been her coping strategy to deal with what has happened to her.*
>
> *John's behavior of avoidance and dismissiveness has signaled her to be wary and disengaged. So even though he is trying to relate to her in this room, her brain is basically telling her to beware.*

Dr. S: Maria, it makes so much sense that you're being very careful. It has to be difficult for you to feel you can even consider letting John in. Can you imagine for a moment that he is sitting here today because he truly wants to be with you, talk to you, and do what we're doing? Can you imagine that?

Maria: Well, I guess I can imagine it, but when I do try to not be suspicious of him, to give him a pass, the minute I am open and vulnerable, he turns away. I really do. I've seen it enough times to know what it looks like.

John: I knew this was going to happen. I just knew that the minute I try to reach her, she gets mad at me and that thing, that cycle, starts all over again. I'm feeling kind of hopeless, like what's the point of coming here. I'm not sure it's ever going to get better.

Maria: There it is. Do you see what I see? Do you hear what I heard? You have to. (Her voice gets more strident.) There is no point to any of this. I came here because I want something different, but he is just a loser. It is too scary to be in life with him because he just gives up on everything when it comes to me and us. I can't live with that. I can't stay with a man who doesn't care enough to try. What is the point? I should just cut my losses now. (Her voice is getting more and more strident, but I see the wetness around her eyes, and I watch her try to wipe away a tear.).

Dr. S: Oh, Maria, the raw feelings that are coming up are filled with so much pain. Pain that comes tumbling out when you hear John speak about his hopelessness. You heard those words of fear and it was just too much, too upsetting. You longed for something different, to matter so much that he'd fight for you, and those words in your mind have convinced you that he just will not be there. You heard his fears say that he was giving up, and it hit you in your deepest place, your heart, which longs to feel cared for, and now you feel frightened, too, that he is giving up on this relationship which feels like he is giving up on you.

Maria: You're right, the last thing I want is for him to give up. It is just too scary, and makes me kind of crazy. It confirms my very worst fears that I don't matter a bit, not at all. All I have ever longed for is to feel that I am worth fighting for, for him to stand by me, and then he just gives up and leaves as if this was just a casual stop in his journey. How can he do such a cruel thing? (Maria weeps again even more.)

John: (He looks at Maria and says nothing for what seems like a very long time.) I don't know what to say. I am completely puzzled. All I have been thinking is that she wanted to leave me, to go back to Italy, and to her good life there. I have continuously felt that I am just not enough for her, and that whatever I have will never be enough. When we first met, I felt pretty special, but now that we're living together here in the US, I've begun to wonder if it's because I am different from her—you know—mixed, biracial, not one kind. I should have been prepared for this. My father warned me that if I got involved with any woman, especially a white woman, this is what would happen. Maybe his warnings are coming true. I always thought it was just because of what happened with my mother, but now I am thinking that maybe he was right all along. I've wondered if she's changed her mind and wishes she were with a white guy, a different guy. So, I have been in a pretty withdrawn state trying to keep out of her way and out of her anger. I felt that the smaller I made myself, the less she'd have to get upset about. I never thought I had a chance with her anymore.

Dr. S: John, you were trying to cope with your fears about being the mate that Maria would want to love and be with. You concluded that this was not possible because you heard her messages as confirming your worthlessness, your difference. Your father's words have come alive, and they feel real. Your internal alarm bell sounded loud and clear, "Get out of here. Don't stay where you are not wanted." And it's also unleashed some real fears, fears that maybe she doesn't feel comfortable with who you are because she sees you differently than when you first met.

John: Well, that's true. I never have believed that I knew how to be a mate. How would I? I was raised by my father who was definitely broken up when my mother left. He's a hard-nosed guy, a military guy, and he pushed me to suck it up and just prove myself. But down deep, I wondered what she'd feel when she came here, living as a mixed-race couple, which is a big deal. To me it's a big deal. You know we never spent that much time together. We had a fun courtship because we lived in two different countries and so mostly it was playing and having fun. But I have always wondered if I was really who Maria wanted or just her ticket to leave Italy and come to the US.

    Hearing myself say this sounds awful, but it has brought up all my racial insecurities. I try not to let that be an issue, but it's there. I figured if she even knew a tiny bit about my deep insecurities, she'd never ever want to be with me. It would seal the deal, and I'd be done. It's not just vigilance. I have never really known where I belong.

Dr. S: You are talking about being afraid of Maria, and her real feelings about you. How difficult it must be to cope with that. To have these scary thoughts and not know what to do with them. Have you ever told Maria about any of these feelings?

John: Told her my feelings about myself? Of course not. I wouldn't do that. I am so ashamed that I feel this way, that this is the way I think. It's so weak.

Dr. S: You think these frightening thoughts so often that—in this way—they do become real. It makes sense that you would try to keep these thoughts out. You were trying to save the relationship by not acknowledging your fears and not saying anything about these feelings. What you are doing here right now is hard. It's hard to deal with what you are feeling right in this present moment, being so vulnerable and transparent. So we need to take this slowly, and respect what is happening to you. (When I looked intently at John, I could see that he looked frozen and stiff.) Maybe your body is talking to you. Our bodies do that, you know. Are you noticing something happening in your body? Can you feel this in your body, on your insides?

John: You're right, this is much more than I was prepared to say. Everything inside me is vibrating, pulsing. I was planning to just sit here and wait it out. I guess what got to me, what makes me come back is that I can't let her say I'm cruel. That is beyond awful. That's not me. She has completely misunderstood me, and I can't let her leave thinking that I don't love her because all I ever did was want to be with her. I just don't know how to get her to believe me, and now I see that more clearly than I ever have before.

> *John is coming out from his silent withdrawn state. But I have no indication that Maria is open to hearing his efforts to connect and care. I don't want to encourage his turning to her when it feels that her walls are still up and reinforced. As long as her system is as rigid as it has been, I don't want to risk emphasizing this pivot that John just made. I have to keep validating his efforts to be more vulnerable and present, to take these enormous risks, and at the same time give Maria the space and regard for why she has to keep herself behind the moat, bolstered and safe. And then there are his feelings about his racial identity. That's such a big piece, and how does he feel with me as a white therapist? I know I need to address this with him, to make space for his concerns, but I need to do this without creating further distance between us. And right this moment, I don't have all the answers. That feels all right for now, but because he's so afraid, maybe he'll expect me to know how to fix everything all at once.*

Dr. S: John, it's hard to risk these feelings, to risk exposing yourself when all you have ever known—what you always learned from your experience—was to keep below the radar without exception. Your body is frantically pulsing because of the awful threat of Maria leaving which you don't want.

John: I am so afraid of that and I don't want her to go.

Maria: Do you actually expect me to believe that he cares about me and whether I stay? You heard what he said before. He accused me of being opportunistic, of using him to come to the US. I am insulted and hurt and feel an even greater need to keep him out. It's just hopeless. There he goes blaming me and making me the bad person. Well, I just won't have this.

Dr. S: Oh, Maria, let's slow down. I hear that you got triggered by John's remarks, and that has set your alarm bell off big time.

Maria: Well, it did. You heard him. He said that maybe I just married him to come to the States. (While saying this, Maria begins to slump in her chair, and she clinches her arms to herself, tears falling like droplets, down her cheeks.) I feel so misunderstood and ashamed. My own husband doesn't know me. He thinks these awful thoughts about me. I am right; I need to leave.

Dr. S: Maria, your heart is feeling such red-hot anger because you believe that John is accusing you of being a user. I know that you two have never really talked about this. And of course, it's been hard for you coming here to a new country where you had to start all over again. From what I'm hearing, you just put one foot in front of the other and trudged on. Sounds like you've been alone with your fears and concerns about all these challenges. And, Maria, you mentioned that this got even worse because of your concern that your agency does not value your work and perhaps there won't be a place for you here. And so you turned inward and John took this as a sign that this was the beginning of the end. John, you withdrew from Maria as well. How awful and alone you each have felt in your own self-created silos.

Maria: I just wanted him to love me and to believe in me. I know I look strong and independent, but I am so much more complicated. And all he seems to notice is the outside me. It does feel cruel—and even dismissive—to just see me that way.

John: I feel so blamed and shamed and I probably deserve it. I've done a terrible job in this relationship as a husband. I've never known how to do that because all I have ever done is work, work, work. That's what I know how to do. I have had to do that, you know, or maybe you don't, but trying to make it in a white world, I've had to push myself all the time. But what I don't know is how to be a husband, and stay with Maria in a different way. I am feeling foolish now for not knowing how to do more. But I can tell you one thing. I want to do more.

Dr. S: John, I hear that you've felt really challenged in the relationship department, and that has been hard. But on top of it, you've also felt that you had to prove yourself, which had to come into play in this relationship, too. I want to make sure that you feel you have a safe place here, but I realize that you're sitting here with two white women, your wife and me. Please help me if at any time I stumble and you feel I am unknowing—like you just did about work—I want to know how you are feeling and if you feel I am getting you. That really matters.

John: I guess you're reading me correctly because I did wonder if you'd be able to understand me. Our differences are a part of all this. My instinct is to be suspicious.

Dr. S: It makes sense that you feel this way but my saying the words isn't going to change this. I know I have to show you in the way I respond and what I say.

John: Nothing has really changed but I do feel better that you're aware of this inequity. I never would have believed that you'd actually know this is part of my experience so this does feel a little bit different.

> *At this point our session was over and I was actually glad that the session was over, even though it had been productive. Both of these lovely people live in a lonely universe. In this session, they each became more vulnerable and present—even though they had not yet turned to each other. This feels right, like we're on a train traveling in the right direction. I would call that having hope, and as a couples therapist, that is something I need to have. I am determined to stay with the process and notice when it moves toward connection. It's not about a specific outcome, it's about becoming flexible and more engaged with each other.*
>
> *Every couple has to find what its version looks like. John and Maria are in the first stages of defining this for themselves. But because of the crises in their connection, they are beginning to notice their patterns and recognize what does not work. This is a positive time in their relationship because they are creating something new that will be*

theirs, based on who they actually are. But of course, at this particular moment, they don't know their way. My role is to help them reflect and make sense of where they are so they can begin to engage about what they want and what they long for in their relationship.

And then there's the question of race. More than ever, I know that it is part of every interaction, especially when there are ethnic differences between the partners—and with me as well. I hope I can help John feel that I want to know his experience. While I can't change my race, I know that being white has the implication of privilege and injustice. I have to listen and be curious and open because undoubtedly there will be missed moments between us. My work is to recognize my part in any issues that happen and try to repair them. Couples work also includes my sensitivity to gender preference, race, and socio-economic considerations that are unique and significant to each unique couple unit.

Later observations of the effect of this session on me: This was one of those times when I could feel the strain in both my being and my body. I get so very tense, particularly in my shoulders. I sometimes wonder if it's like carrying the weight of the pain that exists between these people. I want genuinely to bridge that gap and help them create some connection. But therapy does not stop just because the session ends, and I find myself thinking about what has happened in our session.

I go over what I have done so far and what I regret not doing. I stayed with Maria's painful ambivalent attachment style. I know that whatever has happened, she is wary of connection. She wants to feel good with John but without question believes that doing so is dangerous. She has carried this earlier unprocessed pain into her current relationship and these wounds emerge in moments and times when she gets triggered in her interactions with John. I want to make sure that she knows that I do understand, and more importantly that I am with her. I respect the place that she is in, while at the same time I want her to explore her feelings. That's a pretty big job, and it's the same with John. I can understand and feel for his sense of not knowing what is happening and for revealing his issues about race. He has tried to avoid any emotions whatsoever because they were too dangerous to feel when he was younger. So now he is repeating the same behaviors over and over again, which further signals a dismissive and uncaring stance to Maria.

My goal is for them to see this pattern and be able to give it a name. As long as they continue to be reactive to each other, the conflict will remain the same, as will the feeling of being alone with nowhere to go. This is a desperate state to be in, and I have to hold the course for the time being because they are stuck in the depths of their precariously unresolved relationship.

Chapter 4

Bring on the Addiction

> *I am concerned about the way the last session ended and worried that they will give up coming to these appointments. There was so much despair and hopelessness. Maybe it is contagious, and I'm feeling that way, too. This is hard, hard work, so maybe I am feeling kind of sorry for myself. I need to tell myself to get a grip. I am no different from these people because I am not keeping it together either. (But I put my feet on the ground to stabilize myself and take a moment to briefly recalibrate my nervous system by doing deep inside breathing.) The roller coaster ride is having a vertiginous effect on all of our psyches.*

Dr. S: Maria, I know that we had a very difficult session, and you left feeling that you could not take in John's words. You were so angry with him for what he had done that you continued to feel that there was no way you could turn back. Even with his efforts to talk to you, it felt dangerous and unsafe.

Dr. S: John, hearing your own angry words and verbalizing your thoughts of fleeing made you even more despondent. You essentially turned away with hopelessness. So that cycle of pulling apart was happening again during our session.

It has to be hard to come to these sessions when you feel these painful, desperate feelings, but you know that we're working on being able to heal. That's why I'm wondering what has happened in between our sessions.

John: Well, I was pretty upset last time, and then you asked me about what my body felt like. I never thought about physical feelings, so it was new for me to recognize that my body was really tense. I'm glad you asked me that question because I did pay more attention during the week. I noticed that there was a big difference when I felt that Maria was not so down on me.

Dr. S: That's really good, John. It sounds like you're being more present with Maria. Now, help us understand what signaled you that Maria was not so angry.

John: I just looked at her. I looked in her eyes. And I noticed that they were not so dark and steely. When she is in a bad place, the pupils of her eyes look like lumps of coal.

Dr. S: Like lumps of coal, but they are really hot.

John: Yeah, I can feel her anger through her eyes.

Dr. S: That's right, John, we read our partner's mood and state. These cues are signals that tell where they are, and what their state of mind is like. It makes so much sense that you read Maria's eyes. It's good that this week you noticed—at least on a few occasions—that they were not so fiery.

> 🧠 *I am validating John for noticing Maria's eyes, since he has little sense of what goes on with others. He needs to be able to pay attention, notice, and see Maria more clearly. I am wondering what might have happened in his earlier life that would have discouraged him from considering others feelings. I will have to check with him about his earlier experiences. His coping strategy makes sense because he was an only child of a rigid, angry father. To not be taken over by his father's pain, he blocked out the emotions—and the signals—that were directed at him. Discouraged from tuning into himself and acknowledging his own needs taught him to be wary of others and to concentrate on always being successful. This has become his coping strategy, unconscious but enacted with Maria and others when he becomes unsure and afraid.*

Maria: I know that I do get pretty intense. It has never worked for me to just tell somebody what I feel in a quiet way, so I was pretty angry with John the last time we were here. When we went home, I thought that he'd never talk to me. I was really surprised when he continued to interact.

John: I felt the same way. I expected that you'd just keep yelling at me, and it meant a lot that you didn't do that. I found myself watching you, and assuming that the other shoe was going to fall shortly.

Then I noticed that when it didn't happen, my body started to relax a bit. I feel strange telling you that now. What in the world does that mean?

Maria: Well, I guess I did let up a little bit, but I'm still really concerned about so many things in our relationship. And you, John, had better come clean about the one thing that you know is a huge, huge problem. Tell her, John, about what you do for intimacy. While I was not upset about coming today, I realized I can't go on until we begin to address the biggest problem of all. You haven't been physically close with me. We have no intimacy, almost none. You're on that damn computer all the time. When I come into your room, you try to hide it, but I know what you're doing, and what you are up to. I hate it, and then I start hating you. It's another part of what makes me feel so hopeless because I can't compete with porn and I never will. (Once again, her voice is getting more and more strident.)

Dr. S: Oh, Maria, I hear your painful suffering with feeling bad as well as unimportant.

Maria: You have no idea how awful it's been. I have my own issues with both my body and my inner being, and John's behavior has just sealed the deal. I can't believe that he hasn't understood that. When we first met, he was really into me, and that was all I cared about. I thought it would last, but it didn't.

I've been waiting and waiting for him to remember that I'm here, but his porn addiction has just gotten worse and worse. And this tells me that I'm not worth the effort, and I'm not desirable.

(Maria's head is down, she seems to get smaller and smaller, and her voice is barely audible.)

When I was in University, I was pretty social but I didn't go steady with anybody. I was part of a group and we used to go out dancing and drinking into the night. This was just what we did; everybody did it. One night, we were out very late, and one of the men asked if he could walk me home.

I didn't think anything of it, since this was what we always did. But this time it turned out differently. When I was almost home and we turned a dark corner, he pushed me against the wall, overpowered me, held my mouth closed, and pulled my pants down. And you know the rest. (Sobbing.)

I've never told anybody about this. It's too awful. I feel so full of shame and stupid that I let myself get into that situation. I should've known better, and I didn't. I've never wanted anyone to know. John's lack of interest in me and turning to other women on the internet—has made me feel that I'm a really a damaged person. I thought things were going to be different with John.

Dr. S: Maria, what a terrible experience, and how much you've suffered carrying this all by yourself. It feels unbearable to carry this horror, especially when you're doing this alone. People aren't meant to withstand pain alone, but you felt you had to. You tried to keep going, but it was tearing you up inside.

Maria: Why would I tell anyone? I was at fault, and stupid, stupid, stupid. Everyone knows that you don't go home late after drinking with a strange man. I've tried to put it behind me, but I can't do this now that we're married and my own husband is using porn. It's a clear message to me that I'm not good enough. I think about it all the time, and it's making me crazy.

> *I am watching John's face and he seems so shut down. It's so hard with him as a withdrawer to know what is going on inside. I know that for healing that needs to happen, Maria needs to feel that John gets her pain and really cares that she is suffering. But I don't know if there is enough connection between them for this to happen. I don't want her to turn to him when he's not ready or able to respond. I want to engage him, but not in a way that will leave her feeling that he's cold or indifferent. This is really tricky because he's in a frightened state and still quite guarded.*

Dr. S: John, what's happening inside you? What's coming up for you when you hear about the terrible assault that happened to Maria?

John: I don't know what to say. I'm sitting here, and learning for the first time that Maria is a rape victim, and she never even told me. I'm really upset for her, upset that she had to go through that experience which is unbearable to hear and more awful to imagine. (John pauses for a moment and then blurts out) But I am also feeling marginalized that it took this therapy session for her to bring this up. (His voice became crisp and brittle). What kind of person enters into a marriage and doesn't tell her partner that that has happened to them? I've been feeling that she was pulling away for a very long time. At first, she was really into me. When we would get together, she didn't even want to go anywhere, so sometimes we'd spend most of our time together in bed. Because she was so into me, I began to believe that I was all right in her eyes, and that she really wanted to be with me. But since we've settled into marriage, it is like the light went out. I haven't seen that gleam in her eyes for a very long time. And now I know why.

> *Oh no, Maria reveals a painful wound—a place of shame as well as shakiness—and his first response is a moment of sadness, but then quickly he flips. He becomes defensive going back into his own hurt and rawness, his sense of being excluded, and not important. He's left her alone again confirming that she's correct in not feeling safe to turn to him. How do I manage the pool of pain that fills this room with each of them feeling alone and unlovable? I need to just note the process, and not expect more. They are where they are, and they're coping as best they can—although they may be relying on old no-longer-working strategies. Both partners are in fear states, and believe that the other will not be there. These are their old, deeply held assumptions about others that come from the pain of their lived experiences. When there's anger, and other forms of negativity, they both withdraw. The partner becomes someone to guard against.*

Maria: I knew this would happen, and now it has. Listen to what he is saying. He isn't caring about me or what I have gone through. What he's upset about is that I didn't tell him. He is upset because I brought this up in here with you, and he's mad that it makes him look bad. That's all he ever cares about.

He doesn't care about me. He cares that he looks good in front of you. It's awful, but this is exactly what I always feared. I just knew I didn't really matter, and there it is. It's happening right here in this room for you to see.

Dr. S: Oh, Maria, you've tried to cope with this pain by wanting it to go away. What a terrible experience to go through, and how alone you've been with your shame. When it's inside you this way, there is no place for it to go. Not telling John was a strategy to protect your relationship—and it makes sense. But, in fact, you both suffered. You feared it would change the way he saw you, and now when he says he is upset about not knowing your secret, it just confirms your already-imagined doubts. So, it's a coping strategy that backfired. In trying to protect the relationship, you tried to make the trauma not be there for you, and you could not let John know either. You've been alone and suffering with your pain and sadness.

Maria: I don't know if I can do this, it's too painful. I can't bear him just worrying about himself. It's my worst nightmare.

> *Here it is, the wound that is underneath, the piece that has been between them taking up so much space. Maria is filled with shame and pain that has remained untouched inside of her, and John's behavior has heightened the rawness of this hurt without his ever knowing. I have so much to do, but at least I know what I have to begin with. I have to help Maria deal with her pain, and be able to let John understand what this pain has done to her, and why she needs him to be there. I hope I can do this, but at least I now know what has to be done.*

Dr. S: John and Maria, this room is filled with unprocessed pain. You're each overtaken by the rawness and hurt of what it involves. But I am here with you, and won't let it overtake either of you—not now and not in the future.

What I know is that we have to face these fears together, and that I'll help you do this when we get together in our next sessions. And while it may seem too difficult, please do not talk about this right now. You are learning how to turn to each other, but right now you're not in a place where it is safe. We opened up the conversation about this lack of safety but it's just the beginning. We will be taking time to understand and be with what each of you has been going through.

> *The more I work with this couple, the more confident I feel. It's as if I am gaining my own footing. Of course, that has to happen as I get to know—really know—the individual partners. It's like they become people I can really understand. Ever since I became a psychologist, people have asked me, "So what happens when people are not doing well? Do you just leave the issues behind in the room where you saw them? Does the process go away until you come back together for another session?" In analytic training after my doctorate, I spent a lot of time learning to understand my own reactions to ensure that I checked them at the door so that they didn't interfere with the treatment. This process (called transference) is something that we're all engaged in whether we're in therapy or not. Our experiences and processes—both from our present and our past relationships—are constantly coming into the dynamics with the people who are currently in our lives.*

Transference comes to us like a bolt from the sky. If you've ever experienced a reaction to someone that you're involved with that seems to come out of nowhere, that's the face of transference. There are realms of experience within us that were never encoded in our consciousness. These memories are buried within us, and emerge in these moments to show us that we have lived; it is how we function as human beings. It is the way our brain works. It's as if our mind sees something that we consciously don't really know about, but then—in the present—this knowing registers. Our brain fires, and our emotional alarm bell goes off.

As therapists, we're pretty comfortable with this triggering process because we know it is part of being human. But in some ways, it's a strange phenomenon because it overtakes us when we least expect it.

What I've been feeling with John and Maria is that they are walking in each other's unconscious, untouched experiences, in places they don't even know themselves. If each of them is clueless about what is happening, how can they possibly explain this to their mate? I feel so strongly that I often want to shout out loud, "Transference Time Out. Everyone Stop—you're someplace else with someone other than the person in front of you. Transference is running the show. Don't let it do that. Please silence it once and for all."

Of course, then I'd be the one who'd be out of it, yelling into the void. But I am almost overwhelmed by the process; it feels awful when I am stuck in the middle of this cycle.

I've noticed that if I do some internal self-talk, it helps. But if either one of them is feeling this unknowing, how can they possibly explain this to someone else in the middle of this cycle?

Talking to myself in this way, I can stay somewhat calmer because I know what is happening, and that this is only a moment in the couple's relationship. I also know that I have to help with demystifying what has happened. While I can't do it at the moment, when it happens, I put this in my pocket as something I will bring up later. Being able to think about it that way (and having a plan) helps to stabilize my anxious sense of foreboding. I think about all of this when I'm not in the session because I'm as much overtaken by their process—in some ways—as they are. I think about them when I can stand with each of them separately, and I can feel a great deal of compassion for their struggles. I used to believe that I needed to keep my feelings out of the process, but I don't feel that way any longer.

My job is to know what I'm feeling, and to be able to articulate it as a way to help create more understanding. I have words for my feelings, but am not as overwhelmed as they are. I don't want to influence them in any way, but I attempt to identify and articulate the attachment meaning of the moves they make toward (and away from) each other. This becomes clearer when I'm able to sit with what has happened, and really feel the impact. So, in a sense I carry these people beyond our sessions. I am filled with the pain and fear that is in the room.

Chapter 5

Hopelessness
(Session 4)

This session details the repetitive process of the initial stages of therapy. The couple spends most of their time defending their right to feel what they feel. Whether the partners use words like, "From my perspective," to just stating, "You always," as the therapist, it is necessary to cut through the defensive comments to hear the hurt and fears underneath. Maria's shame of her earlier rape reveals a gaping wound in their partnership. Each needs to feel that what has happened to them matters. John's feelings were hurt because Maria did not tell him about her rape and her secrecy raised doubts for him about being a good enough husband. These fears are played out between them.

> *John and Maria are about to come in. They probably have no idea that on most days, I find myself reviewing the session, and changing my responses because I am unsettled about the way I responded to Maria's disclosure of her rape. To the outside world, when someone has as much training and years of experience as I do, there*

> *may be an assumption that I am certain that I know exactly what I am doing. While I am confident, I also know that I have to constantly and continuously examine the ways I am working, even though it takes a lot of time and energy. I always have considered myself a student, and this is now a part of my process that I feel good about. It's not about doing something wrong, but rather a way of feeling that I am really living the commitment that I have made to my work.*
>
> *Living with my internal process all week, I notice that I am feeling a bit tense right now, anticipating another challenging session. Knowing this, I take steps to calm myself, breathe, and re-center my own nervous system. I do this in order to provide a place where these highly reactive people can begin to recalibrate.*

Therapists are now trained to evaluate their own level of competency. In order to accomplish this, therapists are encouraged to ask for feedback and evaluations from patients on a regular basis. In other words, competency is about being open and seeking to improve and learn. With this as a perspective, when treatment is faltering, competency means recognizing this stalemate and seeking to address this directly with the people involved. Validating the importance of the participant's input further shows respect for the collaboration, which is essential in creating safety and value in the work. Partners have their difficulties, but this transparency remains apart from their conflicts, and in some instances, may affect the outcome by creating a different atmosphere.

Dr. S: Glad to see you back. (I can't help but notice that they are both very glum and quiet, so I reflect on what I see). I am looking at your faces and body language. Please help me know where you are, what you're feeling inside now that you're here.

John: I need to say something. I haven't been able to talk to Maria. Last week she said that the only thing I was concerned about was that I hadn't known about her being attacked and raped. She thinks that I didn't care about what had happened and that I was just upset because I was in the dark, that she didn't tell me about her attack. While it's true that I felt ashamed because I didn't know, what I really was trying to say and I never got it out right, was that I felt terrible for her. It was just crushing to imagine her going along for so long not feeling that she could share this with me. I can only imagine the pain that she had and it's terrible that she had to go through this alone. I couldn't bear hearing that then and even more now when I realize that she did not feel she could come to me.

Maria: Well, I want to hear you, but there's a part of me that still doesn't believe that you really mean this. I keep hearing what you said last week, which confirmed my worst fears, that I really don't matter to you, that I am disposable. I know these are things that I have felt about myself, but you really did a first-rate job in making these fears become real.

    I need you to know more about our getting together in the first place. We never really knew each other. We met and we both needed to have a relationship. We were both speeded up, wanting to connect, wanting to fall in love. There were no brakes whatsoever. We both had our feet on the gas. We were both in a rush to make the fantasy happen. And all that traveling back and forth just made it more tantalizing and exciting. It was like we were on an emotional roller coaster and the excitement made everything seem right. I just knew that I wanted you to see me as perfect and that would make you take me back to the States so I could become the person that I always wanted to be. I was afraid to really let you see me, especially the things that I felt uncomfortable about, ashamed about, wanted not to be there.

John: (John is now looking at Maria, actually looking in her eyes.) Well actually, I did think you were perfect. You are beautiful and smart and you seemed very sophisticated, a woman of the world, speaking several languages and knowing your way around. I figured that you had the courage that I never had. I guess I also hid myself from you, because I believed that if you knew me, if you really saw me, you wouldn't want to be with me, you'd prefer someone else. I have never really fit in or felt wanted by anyone. And of course, lately all you've been doing is talking about going home and how you can't stay. It's like my worst nightmare coming true. I feel so ashamed and worthless. You never sleep with me anymore. I go to bed alone. Even when I try to kiss you, you turn away. Sometimes I feel like I'm a leper, and so what else was I supposed to do? At least when I look at it porn, I feel some satisfaction. I can forget for a moment, the painful feelings that I have.

Maria: There you go again. I heard what you said when you came in the session about regretting that you didn't make your sadness for me more explicit. But listen to you now. I am sitting here and all I feel is that you're blaming me because you are insecure and you didn't feel I was loving you, so you've given up. You haven't been man enough to come to me and let me know what you're going through, you just gave up. How do you expect me to believe that I matter when you just walk away from everything that we've had? Maybe in the beginning I could listen to you when you turned back to me, but now all I hear is you blaming me and complaining about where you are. I really don't feel any empathy for you. I feel hardened and cold and that makes the idea of leaving seem like my only choice.

> *That fear cycle has got these two people in its grip. Her hypervigilance begins immediately when John expresses any pain of his own. When he began to reveal his shame around her not being into him sexually, all Maria could hear was blame, blame, blame.*

Dr. S: Maria, I hear the panic in your voice. I see the tension in your face. I hear your words, and feel your fear. You're broadcasting loud and clear, "Don't come near me, leave me alone." It's like you're shouting, "I don't trust anyone to be near me especially you." PAUSE SLOWLY STATED Please Maria help me know what you're feeling inside when you say those angry words, when you push John away. Please, let's go down inside so I can be with you and the pain. Tell me what you're feeling that's driving those words.

Maria: I feel awful, mortified, and ashamed and I can barely say these words. I am trembling on the inside. Well, you heard him. He's a pornography addict. He gets off on images on the computer which makes me feel absolutely awful. I go to work and when I think about him and what he's doing, I feel like I can't hold my head up among my colleagues. If they really knew what goes on inside my life, they'd think I was crazy to stay with him. What self-respecting woman would stay with a porn addict? I feel so damaged. And when I have tried to tell him about how upset I am, he makes empty promises but never keeps them. So why would I sit here and believe that anything is going to be different, because I know better. I don't want to go through the awful process of believing him, letting him get closer to me again. I did that once, or maybe several times, and then I'm worse off because I hurt even more. It's better for me to just stop feeling for him now.

Porn and Adolescence

There is an epidemic taking over our country. Those most affected are adolescents and young adult males. This condition knows no boundaries. It is not stopped by culture or economic status. It is found in rural America and in teaming cities, on the coasts and in the mountains. It does not know the difference between intact families and those where youngsters are raised on their own. This is the epidemic of porn addiction. Because of the easy access to pornography, John, as with many males, is very susceptible to becoming addicted.

Why is this a phenomenon of our current age? To understand this, we must first look at the brain development of young adolescent males. Biologically their brains are bathed in vasopressin and testosterone, setting in motion their biological ability to ensure the continuation of our species. In the past, this mating urge would be played out in the meeting up with possible partners and learning about them in the experience of being together. But in modern times, there is less physical contact and more involvement by computer-driven devices. And these devices deliver images and situations that are far more stimulating and captivating than any real-life contact. Past generations of men consumed Playboy magazine, looking at the body of a scantily clad young girl. Today, the internet brings these images in rapid order with a frequency and variety that takes over the brain's need for novelty. Increasingly younger and younger boys are turning to pornography. Addiction, as in John's case, may also be a way to regulate painful feelings—to distract when the emotions that are being activated feel unbearable.

Goodness, I have two very frightened people who shut down and withdraw as a way of coping with their pain. They each have tried their own ways of coping, his with pornography, which includes sexual stimulation, an individual way of trying to regulate. Maria uses anger and resentment to close off any of her connection needs, leaving her cold and isolated. Neither knows how to turn to the other to express their longings, needs and fears and believe that someone will be there when they suffer. I need to know more about their earlier experiences because through involvement with family and important others, we develop coping strategies as ways of managing our emotional needs. It's not that these modes of coping are irrevocable, but they have to be understood and recognized for what they are. In this moment I know the work I have to do. I have to stand between these two frightened people and help them begin to look inside themselves, to reflect on their own experience, and make sense of where it comes from and what's getting triggered in the current relationship. But the participants here are both reluctant. Every fiber of John and Maria's pain is poised to withdraw and flee. I have my own fears and trepidations about whether I can hold them to do this work over time. They actually have to become attached to me and feel safe enough to begin the work of self-reflection and emotional processing. But I know the direction I'm going in and what I'm doing. It's like I have a pathway, a road map that I follow. That helps me keep going even when I'm dealing with these massive, reluctant fear states that are pounding down on all of us.

Chapter 6

The Body and Brain in Couples

In our relationships twenty-first century style, partners are often very explicit about their individuality and uniqueness. There is a lot of emphasis on finding oneself and consciously choosing good self-care. Consider the increasing proliferation of online programs for meditation, personal therapy, and various forms of exercise. While independence and self-reliance are important, as mammals we are biologically social beings and as such seek to find and maintain connections to other human beings. We are hardwired to connect. When partners decide to marry or live together, this means having ever constant involvement with the other person's nervous system both positively and negatively. This person becomes the most important person in their emotional universe. From a neuro-psychological perspective, couples serve as emotional regulators for each other and the quality of this process usually determines the state of their relationship, that is, the quality and success of their attachment to each other.

Gender is no longer in the fixed position it once was thought to be. Neuroscience is suggesting it is otherwise. The burgeoning field of the study of our brains shows that fortunately our brains have great plasticity which means that we are likely to have brain changes throughout our lifetime. Initially as infants there is intense dependency on the parent, unparalleled in terms of initial influence. As we grow, multiple influences become important in terms of who we are and who we become. These include and are not limited to: peers, teachers, employers, culture, the environment we live in, and the media we spend our time with. Our brains are affected by all of these factors (Rippon 2019,).

In this narrative, John and Maria are a heterosexual couple. Their responses when under threat should not be considered specific to their gender, but rather in light of their individual predispositions to respond to threats/fear, to cues of danger. These responses would not differ if someone identifies as trans, gay, lesbian, queer, or bisexual. Some, like Maria, become angry and reactive while others, like John, withdraw and shut down. We clearly see this dynamic when changes in John's emotional state threaten Maria's sense of having a secure base in their relationship. Attachment studies show that some individuals tend to be more focused and alert to details of emotional attachment as well as any changes in their relationship. Couples require each other's presence and attention which is not easily available when one partner is preoccupied with unmet emotional or sexual needs perhaps heightened by past trauma. Whether or not these issues are directly spoken about or enacted, the energy and vitality of the relationship is altered by the emotional state of each partner.

How do we explain this pattern from a neuro-biological perspective? Whatever the couple's preexisting attachment relationship, the introduction of trauma or deeply felt rejection destabilizes the attachment bond and interferes with the sense of security and well-being that had previously existed. Couples are very attuned to words or nonverbal cues which alert them to "danger" in their relationship. If the foundation of trust and attachment is insecure, partners can arouse "flight, flight, or freeze" reactions in each other, which are triggered in a millisecond. These reactions occur in the amygdala, an almond-shaped mass of nuclei (mass of cells) located deep within the temporal lobes of the brain. The "amygdala hijack" is an immediate and overwhelming emotional response, often followed by a later realization that the response was inappropriately strong given the trigger. Some emotional information travels directly to the amygdala without engaging the neocortex, higher brain functions. This causes a strong emotional response that precedes more rational thought. In some partnerships, one partner may hold negative feelings both longer and with more conscious attention. This indicates a particular tendency to emotional sensitivity which may result when the reverberations from the shift into flight, flight, or freeze states remain in place longer rather than dissipating as may be the case with the more disengaged partner. This aroused partner does not easily recover from this affective storm. Women have traditionally been thought to be more emotional as opposed to their male partners who are more contained and linear. These differences aren't necessarily based on differences in the anatomical brain but created by differences in the ways males are treated both in their families and in society as a whole. The sensitive emotional processor is more likely to be a careful reader of the expressions on their partner's face. These expressions cue this individual as to the mood and the attachment capability of the partner.

In contrast, the other partner may be less prone to attending to nonverbal emotional signaling and is therefore thought to be less mindful of their partner's state of being. This outward reaction may not reflect the internal state of this more inward person who also may be quite aroused. The more emotional partner is often troubled by this difference in sensitivity and may well take this action personally. Hurt and pain may be explored and redefined as not intentional disregard. It may help to hear about the internal state of the partner that is actually governed by their brain's neuronal process and their actual lived experiences. This dynamic is evident in the interactions between John and Maria.

Our body's regulatory system is disturbed whenever there is intense arousal. When this arousal is not only intense but chronic and frequent, the body's sympathetic and parasympathetic nervous systems respond as if a battle is being waged. Research (Gottman, J. and Silver, M. 2015) has shown that it is the frequency of the hostile complaints (rather than the presence of support) that determines the presence or absence of marital distress. Couples often do not understand how their method of relating may be causing even more dysfunction

Another way of thinking about the differences in partners is found in differences in response to a stressful situation. Taylor and associates (2000) examined the tending behavior that is characteristic of females in a stressful situation. Tending behavior, the instinctual need to care for offspring, is explained as being the neuro-endocrine function that causes the release of oxytocin thought to be necessary in any bonding situation. This pattern of attachment found in early bonding is fundamentally different from the aggression used by some individuals, frequently males, when they are confronted with experiences of threat and danger. The male production of testosterone is thought to be linked to this active aggressive stance. In attempting to avoid the intensity of their feelings, these individuals may shut themselves off by disassociating from their own emotional state. An expressionless face may be an effort to manage an internal maelstrom. Others, often women, may use a similar defense of smiling that is actually an attempt to conceal pain or avoid any conflictual feelings (La France, et al 2003). Couples often end up feeling in direct opposition to each other because of their very different way of responding to a frightening situation. These differences may leave each partner feeling alienated and alone.

Research has shown that pairs co-regulate each other. Humans are dependent on their partners for patterns of sensorimotor stimulation. This includes all forms of communication, both verbal and nonverbal. Partners who are in adversarial states no longer serve as co-regulators for each other, leaving the partner individually vulnerable to experience additional stress and dysregulation. When adversarial patterns become chronic, the relationship as a foundation may become so battered that neither partner is able to recover a sense of stable attachment with their mate.

Couples are constantly reading each other for the signals of attachment or dissatisfaction. As one partner or the other has a negative perception—either actual or created—their limbic system becomes aroused. Our brain's limbic system, located just below the cerebral cortex, is our own internal alarm bell that is in place from the moment we are born. This limbic alarm is a generalist. It registers whether we are safe or not safe; it is not engaged with any conscious thought. At the same time, there are bodily changes in heart rate and muscle tone that may or may not be perceptible to the partner. Again, the more emotionally based partner is generally a more accurate and detailed reader of these changes in posture, flexibility, and facial expressions. Partners in couples therapy often grow up insecurely attached and are dysregulated by too little anger (deadness and detachment)or too much energy (rage, volatility). The right subcortical hemispheres of the partners are not in synchrony, and each feels neither seen or heard by their partner. The couples therapist effectively models right hemisphere attunement, with attention to partners' facial expression, prosody, and nonverbal cues. The couples therapist synchronicity, being experienced by the partners, encourages deeper and more sensitive emotional engagement.

Fortunately mirror neurons inside the brain are activated when someone is seen performing an action or when facial expressions are seen which "mirror" the other's feelings. Mirror neurons allow individuals to bridge the emotional gap between the partners thus making it possible to have empathy for the others. Mirror neurons are very important in allowing partners to experience each other's feelings, thereby identifying and understanding these feelings at a deeper level. Mirror neurons aid the couple in creating new mutual regulation via right-hemisphere attunement.

They underlie and facilitate a couple's ability to change their relationship, and give hope for future of mutual intimacy and positive feelings toward each other. Mirror neurons enable a partner's loving looks and gestures to stimulate a feeling of love and being loved.

Couples may feel that they are destined to repeat patterns that seem impossible to change. They may become discouraged and hopeless about improving their relationship. Fortunately, our brains are capable of "rewiring" or creating new neural pathways that allow all of us to create healthier patterns of relating. Neuroplasticity is a dynamic process that happens within the relationship of mind, body, and brain. In couples therapy, the therapist alerts the couple to dysfunctional patterns of relating and encourages more rewarding patterns. The lived experience of more rewarding and sensitive responses from one partner allows the other partner to risk responding in a different and healthier way. The repetition of new ways of relating—within and outside of therapy—establishes new relationship patterns that can strengthen the couple bond. New ways of relating within couples therapy can also create a "butterfly effect" in which small changes can be the catalyst for larger changes in the couple relationship. The couples therapist acts as a temporary attachment figure providing safety and focus so these new patterns can be practiced and observed.

The therapist becomes an attachment figure by demonstrating aspects of relating that are felt to enhance and contribute to the relationship. The relationship John was developing with the therapist highlights several of these conditions. Knowing that John is biracial, the therapist recognized that their racial difference could be a potential problem between them. Their interaction over several occasions showed that the therapist began to directly address and reassure John that he was safe and accepted for who he is. By attending to this issue, she showed that she has the capacity for empathy. If the therapist did not feel comfortable and felt little interest in John's well-being, these subtle yet dismissive feelings would have seeped in and corroded their relationship. This interaction cannot be seen in isolation. But something began to change in that John indicated that this conversation was unusual for him. The unexpected or novel is worth noting.

Why would this experience, this small moment, be helpful in building the connection to the therapist? The therapist's ability to express and demonstrate consideration and caring was lived and enacted. These are the moments that inform John about the therapist's ways of being, of the actual way she treats others. If clients have had parental figures who are not consistent and have suffered from their own unprocessed fears, then like John, such individuals have ways of avoiding connection to others. Even the therapist can be seen as someone potentially dangerous, someone to guard against. This is not to suggest that this interaction will cause a fundamental change in John. On the other hand, one never knows for sure what causes another human to change their feelings, so the therapist's holding a consistent, thoughtful stance is what John will experience in various ways and in multiple experiences. The therapist is grounded in relating to John continuously reflecting what she believes in: her commitment to know and walk with John in his inner world.

Watching John and Maria's struggle, we see the process of dysregulation come alive, with the resulting amygdala hijack occurring all too often. Their mutual intrapsychic rigidity makes it difficult for them to change course. The therapeutic process of slowing their arousal down, alerting them individually to their own unique response, is the pathway to developing emotional flexibility. Instead of falling back on their habitual ways of coping alone, they are learning they can turn to each other to get through difficult times and experiences—the fundamental basis of feeling more secure. This experience, repeated over time, can create new neuronal pathways and hence feels different. The sympathetic nervous system is calmer and no longer in an aroused, reactive state. Right hemisphere attunement within the triad (therapist, John and Maria) allows greater sensitivity and affect synchrony (Lapides, 2011).

Effective couples therapy alters more than the left-lateralized conscious mind of the partners. It can also influence the growth and development of the partners' unconscious "right mind." Although both brain hemispheres contribute to effective therapy, in light of the current relationship trend that emphasizes the primacy of affect, the right brain (the social emotional brain) is dominant in all forms of psychotherapy and therapeutic attunement (Schore, 2014). We will be seeing this attunement unfold as the sessions with John and Maria progress.

Chapter 7

Slow Down and Listen
(Session 5)

Maria and John are continuing to repeat their dance, their pattern of disruption and withdrawal from each other. We can imagine that by moving to America, becoming an immigrant, and feeling a loss of professional status, Maria has become increasingly insecure. She attempted to seek reassurance from John but to him it felt like blame. He felt rejected and read her emotional signals as her way of telling him to go away.

As with many protesters, Maria's pain turned to anger when she felt unnourished. In this encounter, the therapist is trying to heighten the withdrawer signals of distress so that Maria will soften and engage once more.

> *Another challenging session. I find myself anticipating having to deal with disruption and pain. This is not good. I should not be starting out in this state of mind. I am bringing my fears into the mix and that is not all right. I will have to see how I am doing. I wonder if I should seek a consult about my concerns and worries. There is a*

> *misconception that as a seasoned therapist, I have complete confidence and know what I am doing at all times. It is more important that I know when I am being pulled into the couple's conflict and about to lose my way. I am not there yet with John and Maria, but a consult might help stabilize my work with them.*

Dr. S: I want to check in with how you are feeling.

Maria: I'll go first. I am still feeling pretty hopeless about our connection and the future. I can't go on much longer. I look at John and don't see anything that makes me feel that he truly cares. This is happening right now in this session.

Dr. S: Oh, Maria, you said that when you look at John, you can't see anything that gives you hope. I see you looking at John. Can you help me with what you see in John's face that's making things so difficult and stuck for you?

Maria: There's no expression in his face. His eyes look flat and kind of distant. I don't see any interest in them and it makes me want to close up and go away. I don't know why I bother to tell him. There's no point. He doesn't care.

> *Oh, I feel the pressure for this woman. She's so tender, tentative, and ambivalent about trusting. There are many reasons why that is so, and in this moment, her husband's lack of emotional engagement sends the message to her that she's right about being wary and guarded.*

Dr. S: John, did you have any idea that Maria is watching your face for signs of your interest in what she is going through? Because of her connection to you, she's literally reading your face and your eyes.

📋 Non-verbal cues

An important role of couples therapists is helping couples "read" each other's nonverbal messages and learn that they are bombarding each other with these messages whether or not they are conscious of it. Important cues are found in facial expression: including eye rolling, clinched teeth, averting one's gaze, and failure to make eye contact. Any of these behaviors may be indicative of the avoidance of anger and other strong negative feelings. So many nonverbal messages occur in a millisecond and register at a subliminal level. Our brain, specifically the limbic system, is superb at registering nonverbal cues indicating danger. This alerts the nervous system to react: to fight, flee, or freeze.

Humans have communicated with each other since the beginning of time. The brain has used the cues that it picks up such as tone of voice, cadence of the vocalization, body language and hand gestures, and the expressions transmitted through the eyes as part of this communication. No matter what language is used, these modes of communicating feelings have existed across centuries and know no geographical or social boundaries.

In our modern world, in our often-distracted, overstimulated environments—even in intimate relationships—we may not process the person's emotional state that is often quite evident in their ongoing communication. In this narrative, John and Maria expectantly watch each other carefully for nonverbal signs of anger and disinterest, instead of love, interest, and approval.

Notice that Dr. S points out that Maria is watching John's face for signs of interest and caring. John is surprised that he is important enough that she would study his facial expression. This is a turning point for the couple as they are confronted with a possible new experience.

John: I never knew I was that important to her. She's reading my face and my eyes. She's looking at me to see what's inside. I never thought about that. She always seems so self-contained and self-assured, I just figured that she can do without me.

Maria: (Her face getting a little tense and her eyes again becoming a bit fiery . . .) Are you kidding, John? You know how much I need you! I told you that and you never seem to listen or care. I feel like I've always been waiting for you, waiting for you to be interested in me. Waiting for you to pay attention to me. And what I know is that I'm just supposed to be there when you want me to be. Otherwise, I don't feel that you care. I'm just a function in your life. This is especially true in terms of our sex life. I have to service you and that's about it.

> *So now they've laid out their cycle—the way they pull apart based on the pain they each feel in terms of their connection. I need to help each of them to understand their part of this distress, but that can't happen when they are withdrawn in self-protective modes. John feels her criticism and dissatisfaction and has shut her out. Earlier in their relationship, Maria was engaged in wanting John's attention, but when she felt he did not understand what she was going through, she withdrew*

> *from the relationship, fueled by anger and resentment. They are both in intense, unspoken withdrawal from each other.*

Maria: I know I brought my problems to this relationship, but John just wants me to be there when he wants to have sex with me, which is not very often. After this happened so many times, and he's not trying to understand my emotions or feelings, I've kind of turned off and decided that there's just no point. I have to keep this to myself because he's not interested in me or how I feel.

Dr. S: So, you took his distance as a sign that he doesn't care. And it sounds like you've pretty much shut down and withdrawn.

Maria: What else could I do? Why would I put myself in a position to be disappointed and hurt again?

Dr. S: That makes sense, Maria. It makes sense that when you have tried to signal John of your need and you felt that he didn't get it, you've coped with this rejection by just giving up, by withdrawing to protect your heart from any more pain.

Dr. S: (John's head is down and he has closed his eyes.) John, can you tell me what's happening with you right now? I see your face and I just want to touch you and help you with what's happening inside you. Would that be all right?

John: (Barely audible . . .) I know that I usually don't listen when Maria says these things to me because I can't stand hearing how bad I've been. I want to stop her complaints because there is nothing that I can tell her to defend myself. I just feel bad about everything.

Dr. S: Oh, John, it's hard when you have these sad feelings. But they're part of being a human being and you're feeling something about the woman you love even though you feel distant from her. Being sad when you feel the loss of someone you love makes so much sense. Maybe Maria has read this sadness as disinterest and had her own reaction to that, believing you no longer cared about her. You each saw in the other's actions which have meaning to you. And what you saw is about loss and abandonment.

John: You're right. At this moment I feel like I can say that I feel bad about Maria's pain. I've never felt that I could let her know this because of all I've done. My lack of response was never because I didn't care. Never—not ever!

Dr. S: I know you care. I can hear and feel it. Can you help us know what your heart is saying when it hears Maria's words?

John: My heart hurts to hear her distress but my head keeps telling me not to let the awful, dark feelings in. That's why I withdraw and shut her out. I know I am a master at that. I've always done my best to make those awful feelings go away because these words are coming from the person who matters most to me, my wife. I learned this lesson early on because I was constantly feeling that I disappointed my father. I wasn't the tough, black son that he wanted and expected.

Dr. S: John, that makes sense. I hear how your instinct is to protect yourself, to shield yourself from even more pain. You've tried to do everything not to experience the terrible feelings that are taking you down. Am I getting that right?

John: You sure are. I had to do that. I had to make sure that I didn't let anything get in because I was always expected to just do it right and sometimes, I couldn't do it. And I couldn't bear disappointing anyone, so I couldn't let myself feel anything about any situation that wasn't working.

> *I am glad that this is happening, but it sure is hard to be with. John is being quite vulnerable. I need to validate his courage to be present. He is laying out how he has learned to cope by not letting anything in—by not feeling anything at all. And, of course this was necessary because he did not have anyone who was involved in understanding what he was going through. This makes sense when I think of his father trying to raise him while in the military as a single father.*

In this chapter, there are examples of those fractal self-repeating patterns which cause frustration for both the couple and the therapist. Maria feels disappointed by John's withdrawal from her, and John withdraws more because he cannot bear hearing how he disappoints Maria over and over.

The therapist identifies this pattern, naming it as it occurs and making it possible for the couple to begin recognizing their repetitive pursue-withdraw pattern. Recognizing their "dance" is the first step for partners in changing this self-repeating pattern which ultimately affects the feelings of each partner about their relationship.

CHAPTER 8

IMPLICIT TO EXPLICIT
(SESSION 6)

In this chapter, John and Maria continue in their pattern of disengagement and withdrawal. If that seems repetitive, it certainly is. We notice that in this partnership, as long as the dynamic brings up familiar feelings such as resentment and anger, the conflict continues. Most couples talk incessantly about the external conditions that cause them to be upset. And usually this leads to blaming the other person. John and Maria have issues with their differences, including sex, which is addressed in this session. The shift in their ability to communicate comes when each begins to reveal their inner experience, their deeper feelings about themselves, and what they experience internally, deep inside while these feelings are coming alive. These signals of pain and distress alert the partner of the deep suffering and needs for caring. These are the messengers that cue the partner to begin to feel empathy and concern. We can see the beginning of this process as we follow John and Maria in their next session.

The Roller Coaster of Emotion

> *Maria and John are coming back today. I'm aware of feeling tension emotionally and physically. This couple came into treatment without a firm foundation, and they have given me the task of helping them build one. That is absolutely essential, but their situation is evocative because it has been on shaky ground since the beginning. How do I foster their courage to face their fears with each other, and to become vulnerable with each other? It's the only way for them to begin to walk in life together rather than retreat and withdraw.*

Maria: I notice that even after five sessions, John continues to show up even though I've blamed him and said some pretty bad things to him in here. I don't want him to think that I don't notice what he's doing. I do see it. I guess I can't just keep saying that he doesn't care, but that's what it feels like most of the time. It is especially upsetting because of his porn addiction. When I think of him doing that, looking at the computer screen and pleasuring himself, it sickens me. It makes it impossible for me to feel close to him. I wish he'd understand and change his behavior, because it's just too painful to believe that it will get better when it happens again.

Dr. S: Oh, Maria, it's like you gave your heart to John believing that he will care for it, but then it happens again, and he seems to drop it. It must feel like he forgets that you are there trying to connect. That's the pain, the awful letdown, and so it's like you have to vow—to promise yourself—to never let him in, or to let him matter again.

Maria: You got it. That's really the way I feel. It's why I have my walls up, and why I keep coming here to tell you what he's done. I can't stand myself when I sound so negative, which is another part of the pain. I can't bear seeing myself and what all of this has done to me. I'm becoming someone I don't like. I've turned into a blaming shrew, an angry woman. I used to think of myself as someone who was loving, and I used to like myself but now this has changed. Today, I can barely look at myself because I am so annoyed and angry most of the time. I feel dark inside and kind of hopeless. It's like the windows have venetian blinds that are permanently closed, and there's not even a cord to open them.

Dr. S: That makes sense, Maria. It feels safer to close the blinds and throw the cord away because the hurt from the disappointment is too much to bear. You keep wanting John to hear that the light has gone off in your heart and in your being. You feel dark and changed, and you don't like it. You keep broadcasting and signaling this message to John so that he'll come forward and wake up. But it feels like he's asleep, like he's thrown the keys away, shut his eyes, and closed his heart to you. That feels awful.

Dr. S: John, what's going on inside your heart as you are listening to Maria's sense of despair and futility?

John: This feels like all that I know. Maria keeps telling me what a loser I am. She's so dismissive and full of rage. I feel like I lose my manliness when I stand in front of her. I feel like a skeleton, an empty body. I'm mostly detached from myself, and feel that I have little worth. This has become unbearable. At least when I watch porn with couples having sex, I don't feel this terrible searing pain. I discovered this escape one night over a year ago. Ever since then, I distract myself to keep from experiencing those awful feelings by looking at these other people engaged with each other. I can feel the sensation of pleasure when I give myself permission to watch them. It's pretty awful, isn't it? But at least it's better than feeling the emptiness and loneliness that have become a big part of my life.

As I watch John talk, I notice that his voice gets softer and softer as he describes his masturbatory experiences when he watches pornography. I'm aware that this man is becoming more vulnerable than he ever has been before just by staying in this room and talking with his mate about his way of "regulating" himself with pornography. I hope that she is hearing this, but I see her staring straight ahead. I wonder what she's thinking. Has she already left the room because of what she's hearing from her mate? I have to help her bear what she's feeling without being overreactive. Based on what I've seen before, that's going to be hard.

Maria has a high-arousal nervous system, which means that when she has a feeling, she reacts to it immediately and then broadcasts it. When she's uncomfortable or distressed, she immediately wants to communicate her need to feel that someone is there to notice and care about what's happening to her. The clinical term that could be applied to Maria would be "anxious and ambivalent." But those words really

> *don't explain what's underneath and why this behavior makes sense for this person. Maria is exhibiting a deeply engrained need to feel cared for, which causes her to pursue and demand. Maria is afraid of not getting what she needs. She is vigilant to either make sure that John cares about her, or reacting to a felt sense of not mattering. This wounding can occur in the most ordinary moments. I have to help her to comprehend this, and supply words to her own behavior.*

📔 *One of the main tenets in couples therapy is to make the implicit, explicit. That means we give words and explanations for the processes that go on in the partnership. Why does this matter? Because as humans we know that we generally function much better when we are aware of what we're doing and how it affects us. That is an integral part of the therapeutic space and experience that is separate from everyday life. Each person can sit with his or her inner feelings and begin to be curious about these thoughts and how they affect the relationship. That is what is happening right now, and why I feel good about John's revelations even though Maria is still withdrawn.*

Maria: If I really tell you how I'm feeling, it frightens me. I know I'm supposed to feel empathy for what John's talking about, but I'm not there yet. I'm committed to what we're doing, so I'll be totally honest that listening to him describe his emptiness and feelings of worthlessness is too scary for me. I grew up when my father died, and when that happened, it was as if the life that I once knew stopped forever. I had no one to go to. I was left with my mother who was so anxious and afraid that she basically left me alone to manage myself and cope with what I was going through. There was literally nobody home. And that's what it feels like to me when John expresses his vulnerability. He may be seeking closeness, but I just feel more distant. And now I'm back being the little girl with a dead father and a widowed, anxious mother.

Dr. S: Maria, I hear you digging into your feelings, going inside and touching the pain that is keeping you where you are. That's hard to do when it hasn't worked before, and it takes a lot of courage to be here in this space and do that. Have you ever let John know when you're feeling that inner pain of trusting and being in this relationship?

Maria: I don't talk to him that way. I just assumed that he wishes I'd be happy—which I am not—and that he doesn't want to know what I am feeling. As a result, I feel angry a lot of the time, and that's what he hears. I can see that being angry is what I am used to, and I know now what this has caused between us. I really didn't know how to do anything else. Everybody I've ever lived with and been close to has behaved this way. Everybody I know has blamed the other person when they feel lonely or upset, so I just thought that that's the way to get my feelings across. It seems so simple here, but I've never known how to do it.

Dr. S: Maria, can you imagine sharing this pain with John, and letting him know that you've longed to feel that he cares about what has happened to you? Can you let him know about your deeply felt yearnings?

Maria: I can imagine, but I also worry that he'll come back with a rejection. Why wouldn't he, when I've been so awful at times? That's what I am feeling now—shame for having been immature. I should have known better, but I didn't.

(Maria turns to John . . .) I am sorry that I have been so out of control. I have felt like I was all alone in a raft drifting out to sea, and that you didn't even care if I was gone.

In this moment in the treatment, Maria dares to come closer by stating her needs. John, revealing his relational fears, retreats into his familiar—but painful—repetitive pattern of labeling himself a "loser." Maria pursues and John withdraws. But the softening of his voice and his vulnerability signal some readiness to risk venturing out from his familiar withdrawal pattern of coping. John and Maria are having a new experience with the therapist who is holding both of them by acknowledging their fears. Knowing that the therapist is there to assist both of them with new attachment behavior and new self-organization is essential for their change.

John: I do care. I care more than you know, and I feel awful that you've been hurting so much for so long. I've wanted to come to you so many times, but I always saw you as not wanting me, and not really needing anything.

You seem so confident and self-assured, so what I am left with is feeling really inessential and unimportant. I've longed for it to be otherwise, but things always happen that make this awful situation seem like a grim glimpse of what the future is going to be. We never have sex anymore even though I've made so many advances toward you and tried to interest you in every way possible. I've told you that this is my language of love, but it doesn't seem to make any difference. You always have an excuse as to why you are too busy or just not available. What else am I supposed to conclude except that you are not into me, and that my body and being just don't matter to you? I try to remember the way it was when we first met, but that was so long ago, and things were totally different between us then.

Maria: (Her face getting tense and tight . . .) I knew it. There you go again blaming me for all our troubles. You say you care about me, but then within a millisecond you are complaining about my behavior and what you call my limitations. I think you are just waiting to tell me how bad I am, and that this awful situation is all my fault. In your eyes, I can't do anything right. When I came in today, I knew that it was just hopeless. My instinct was to turn away and get out. Now I feel that in all of my body. I don't know what I expected in the first place. Apparently, I live in a fantasyland.

> *John tried to signal Maria about his longing, but it did not go anywhere. What she heard instead was that their situation was a mess, and that she was the culprit being blamed for everything that went on between them. Maria has spent her life trying to make sure that she does things correctly, and because of this way of coping, it is as*

> *if she is feeding an insatiable beast. Aware of her early experience, I feel like I am walking with both her and her mother—the anxious parent who felt overwhelmed much of the time.*
>
> *Maria's brain is wired to make sure she's doing everything right, that she's where she needs to be. It's as if her brain is telling her: "If you want to be loved, you have to keep the object of your affection completely happy. But even if you try your hardest, it will never be enough. Who do you think you are?" Can you imagine living this way? No wonder Maria began to withdraw, close off, and feel frightened of ever really mattering. I have to help these good-but-scared people begin talking about what is really going on with them, as well as the fear and shame that is lurking so close to the surface.*

John: She's so intent and convinced that I don't care about her or have any real interest. I tried and tried to get her to want me sexually, especially when we finally got settled and began to live our lives. I told her repeatedly that I would be fine as long as we could have physical contact. I didn't care much about how I got it as long as she was at least recognizing my need. I'd be satisfied with a kiss, a hug, a touch, a caress, or anything that would show that she wanted to be close and feel me. When she does that—even if only a few times—it reassures me, calms me down, and gives me a feeling that I matter.

Dr. S: I hear that you feel like you've let Maria know this, but that it didn't make any difference.

John: Difference? She's been indifferent whenever I have tried to let her know how I feel about this. She'd be present and involved for a short time, but then she and I quickly start slipping away from each other. We were together physically, but I knew she was not into me anymore. I just have not known what to do. I want to be with her and to have her care for me, but all I ever feel is rejected. It's like I am an annoyance that must be avoided. That's why I have kind of given up.

You've heard about my porn use. Well, at least I can count on the images being there. I control them, and when I am involved, that's something that really matters to me. I need to feel as if I have some control over what is happening to me. Life with Maria is like being on a perpetual roller coaster because I never know where she is emotionally. I was probably attracted to this part of her before, but now it is so lonely, and impossible to bear. Especially now, since she is constantly talking about returning to her home and family.

Maria: He thinks he's communicating to me about this, but I'd hardly say that yelling at me about how ungrateful I am is talking to me about his feelings. All I know is that he blames me for our problems sexually, and when I have that feeling, it makes me so angry about being unjustly accused that I want to go out the door and away from him. I kind of feel that way now. It's hard for me to be here and sit with these feelings.

Dr. S: I hear what a big deal this is, and how hard you have to work to stay engaged here. Especially when every fiber of your being is telling you to run the other way. Is that what your voice inside is saying?

Maria: You are on the mark. Every part of me is on hyper alert. It feels dangerous in here. My gut is telling me to just get out, not to engage, and definitely not to trust.

Dr. S: Maria, you're letting me know that you are in high distress. Your brain and all your bodily systems are firing the signal, Danger, Danger, Danger! That happens when the person we are closest to makes us feel frightened. Almost as if he or she is kind of like an alien—essentially, a person we don't know.

With John, it's hard because when you feel his unhappiness, it sets off your alarm bell of doing something "wrong," which is a place that you try to avoid. When you feel unjustly accused, your defenses are heightened and you pull away, which signals to John that his efforts to connect are in vain. So now both of you are frightened, overwhelmed, and withdrawn from each other. It is as if you are both in the ocean in a storm, and while you can see each other far away, there is no way to connect. It feels both overwhelming and hopeless.

Maria is experiencing a strong limbic system reaction. Her amygdala is sending her "fear messages" and urges to "flee the danger" she is experiencing. She literally has an internal alarm bell warning that his behavior is dangerous, and may have disastrous consequences. In their couple relationship, both Maria and John have strong fears of rejection and abandonment. When these fears are engaged, avoidant

> *behaviors also become activated. Paradoxically, this heightens the possibility of loss. This repeating pattern can be very difficult to change.*

We have learned from neuroscientists that the part of brain known as our limbic system is the seat of our emotional regulation. While we are unaware of its existence, this part of our body, the actual apparatus and structure we are born with, is involved in everything that happens to us. Whether a small moment or a major event, these experiences are processed in some way by our brain's system. The primary player in this processing is the amygdala, which is registering in the most general of ways, whether or not we are safe. In this sense it seems accurate that experiences sculpt the basic form of our brain. What we know is that there is no such thing as a fixed brain. The general pattern of experience shapes how the brain responds. Simply put, is the world safe or not safe, or in relational terms, are others safe or not safe?

Let's consider how understanding how the brain works relates to John and Maria. These individuals are perfect examples of people who have highly reactive emotional systems. When we first met them, they were mutually reactive to each other. In clinical terms, they were unable to engage in limbic resonance. When we are attached to another person, there is frequent right-brain to right-brain communication; it occurs spontaneously and rapidly when the two people are emotionally engaged. You have heard people say something like, "She was there and talking but she really wasn't "with me." The speaker is talking but the partner is not feeling the other's presence or engagement. When a person is in limbic resonance, their brain is in sync and able to read the emotional state, the inner world of the other person, their partner. John and Maria were in great distress because neither felt safe and cared about by the other. They are exhibiting limbic distress. Part of therapy, especially couples therapy, is to increase the emotional engagement, the limbic resonance.

Maria: You are right. I am hopeless, and I do want to withdraw. What's the point, why should I stay? I have needs, but he doesn't care. It is just like when I was a girl, alone in my family, where no one had a clue about how much pain I was in.

> *I am breathing a sigh of relief because she is finally touching both the deep pain and the unresolved terror that became part of her experience. It is good that she is beginning to slowly unpack this with John.*

Dr. S: Tell us more, Maria, about this well of pain and hurt that is coming up now.

Maria: When my father died, all of us were in mourning, but in some way, I lost my mother, too. She had no idea about how deep and unbearable my feelings were at that time. My father was my rock, my guide, and my supporter. The world felt like an empty place after he died, and I did not relate to my mother at all. In fact, I felt like I had to make her feel all right by keeping up a front and looking all right. I resented her deeply for this, and so whatever I felt just went deeper and deeper inside me. That's what I still do whenever I feel anything critical about myself and my inner experience. I suppose I have done it with John, too. I have believed and been afraid that if he knew my inside thoughts, he'd disapprove or judge me, and see me as bad and selfish.

Dr. S: Bad and selfish?

Maria: For sure. I believed that a good person just felt content all the time, and never had an unhappy or angry thought about anything. So, when John wanted sex, I'd just go along with it, no matter when and no matter what else I was doing. I'd check my feelings and wants at the door, and accommodate him. It wasn't that way at first, but his appetite is different from mine, and so I didn't dare let him know my true needs. I just showed up and went along, but I didn't really want to be there.

Dr. S: You kind of checked out and withdrew into yourself more and more.

Maria: I did that, for sure. And I did it for a very long time. I guess that is why I began to essentially give up on our relationship. I figured that if I was going to be so alone, I'd be better off moving back home where at least the culture is more familiar, and I have a strong support system from my friends.

Dr. S: John, what's happening inside your heart? Did you have any idea about the depth of your partner's fear and pain?

John: I am overwhelmed. Since we have been coming here, I now realize so many uncomfortable things that it is almost more than I can bear. Maria, I had no idea that you were so uncomfortable and felt so marginalized. I hear that now, and it feels awful, absolutely terrible. I felt your lack of energy and interest, but I assumed it was because you had given up on me and on us. That you were afraid to talk to me because you believed that I'd just minimize you is horrible. Because my mother left and did not try to see me, I have always carried the fear that her rejection would repeat itself if I became emotionally involved with a woman. And my father drilled into me the motto that I had to protect myself with everyone. My horror was that I began to see this pattern with us when I could not get you to come back to me. Maria, I feel truly ashamed and sorry for all of this, and the effect it has had on you.

> *Oh, my goodness, am I hearing this for real? Listening to John begin to turn and talk to Maria gives me such a good feeling. When I hear something like what John is saying about his seeing and feeling remorse for the first time, I experience an amazing sense of relief. Even though I know intellectually that this process works, it is really something to watch it happen in the session. Moments like this, the possibility of repair, deepen my connection to this work. And I hold these moments to offset discouragement when the healing process is stuck or headed in the opposite direction.*
>
> *I feel hopeful that this couple may be able to make their way through the challenges that have been affecting them. John has begun to communicate that he recognizes his part in the dynamic that has existed between them. Now, I need to do a good job of helping them understand how this has interfered with their ability to be happy with each other.*

The Roller Coaster of Emotion

Dr. S: John, you're picking up on those signals that Maria is sending. You are beginning to hear her pain and acknowledge her attempts to let you know that she has been in a very dark place and felt unable to let you know. You are recognizing your own anxiousness, too. Can you touch this and go a little deeper?

John: Well, I'm sitting here listening to her talk about her long-ago need to not make any trouble when she felt how distressed her mother was. You know, I came from a family where there was divorce. I'm an only child, and I was aware of everything that was going on. I felt incredibly responsible to keep things in a good place. My parents divorced when I was around seven. They had never had a good relationship, so it was no surprise. I had wondered when they would stop being with each other, even though I didn't know exactly what that meant. I just knew that I hated the noise that I heard each night when they'd yell at each other and have these horrible fights. We lived on a military base, and my mother wanted out of there. At first, I saw her, but then after a while she moved away, got married, and made a new life elsewhere leaving me with my father's anger and unresolved feelings of rage. He basically became an alcoholic, so I learned to watch and to try to keep away from anything that would make him angry. I became preoccupied with remaining under his radar.

Dr. S: Oh, John, how hard for you to navigate such a treacherous course. How hard to feel scared of the person who is taking care of you. Clearly, you suffered because of this. I can only imagine how alone you must have felt with the sense that you had to keep on going in spite of all of that was going on in your home.

John: It's weird to hear you use the word suffer. I've never thought of it that way. I guess I felt so ashamed of the way I felt about my father. I know he tried to raise me to be a productive person, but he really didn't know me at all. I've always wanted to keep as far away from him as possible and so I kind of raised myself. When my mother stopped being involved with me, I had to make her not matter, too. I've never wanted to tell anybody about this because it feels positively crazy. Almost like something out of a movie.

There it is. Each of these good people is finally explaining how they learned to cope. Maria and John have both experienced themselves as responsible for their parents' emotional states, and they both have experienced traumatic loss. I need to be able to link this in a way so that they can begin to understand the dynamic that exists in their dance together as a couple. Clearly, they are both carrying enormous pain that has to be brought into this room so it can be dealt with safely. As I sit and listen to them, I feel that they have no understanding about the connection between their earlier relationships and the ways they are behaving toward each other. Part of the therapeutic process is to help people find ways to think about what is going on in their relationship. This includes being able to name their feelings and see them as reasonable responses to their lived experiences. This normalizes their situation, which in and of itself can help calm the reactivity that has often become part of fearful emotional states.

Dr. S: Maria, what is coming up inside as you listen to John's feelings about what you said?

Maria: Well, in some way I feel a little more like he's trying to hear me. At least I don't feel quite so much as if I'm being blamed. I do know, however, that I've been in this very angry place for a long time, and hearing this today doesn't take away from what I've felt like over this past year. I'm glad we're sitting in this room with you because I know we have a lot more to talk about. I don't feel safe with him yet, or as if all my concerns have just been taken away. Maybe it's because—as it was in my childhood—my mother would be all right for a while, but then something would snap and she'd become depressed again. That would signal me that I needed to stay there and do exactly whatever she needed. It wasn't like she was mean or anything, but she was so pathetic, so helpless. I just knew that if I wanted to be something in my own life, I had to make sure to never be like that. I couldn't let her affect me because I knew it would slow me down.

Dr. S: Maria, that makes so much sense. You learned to turn off the cues that your mother was emitting because they were keeping you from going on in your life. Seeing someone else's pain was a dangerous thing, and it could make life impossible for you.

Dr. S: We have a lot to talk about when we get together again. Did you notice what happened today when you began to talk to each other? You both have done such a good job today with being able to slow down and actually listen to each other. You began to relate to your earlier experiences, which have a lot to do with how you have learned how to cope. That's what happens to all of us as we learn about how to be with others from our experiences in our earlier relationships. We are going to stay in the present, but it helps a lot if we can also pay attention to what may be coming up inside you about your past. It is all part of what is going on here and now. I hope this is all right for you. (Both nod yes, so I am relieved.)

> *Effective couples therapists "carry" and convey hope for the couple's ability to change. The couples therapist's hope, curiosity, and interest are felt by the couple via our emotional brains (the limbic system). Also, when the therapist notices "small changes" in the couple's relationship, it helps to heighten their awareness regarding their mutual ability to create a new structure of self-repeating patterns.*

CHAPTER 9

COUPLES AND PATTERNS

Being part of a couple is a goal that most of us have from a very early age. The rhyme, "Johnny and Jenney, sitting in a tree, k-i-s-s-i-n-g. First comes love, then comes marriage . . ." is commonly known and frequently repeated on playgrounds. The next part of the rhyme, ". . . then comes ____ with a baby carriage," is said with glee and giggles as our biological instincts to mate and reproduce are implied. In this rhyme, one step leads seamlessly to another: kissing to love to marriage to baby. It symbolizes how being in a couple relationship is prized in our society. Once a mate is chosen there is the hope that they "will stick like glue" together. When a couple bond is seriously threatened for any reason, couples become anxious and can enter a flight, fight, or freeze state. When this occurs, couples often reach out to a couples therapist for help.

As in the linear playground rhyme, for many years the primary concept about how relationships occur and change was linear: one thing causes another to change in an orderly fashion. Linear thinking was also predominant in psychotherapy: the therapist makes a brilliant interpretation or meaningful statement to her patient and the patient changes their thinking and behavior. But how we view change in psychotherapy has evolved to dynamic, systemic, and complex thinking. We realize that life is not orderly or step-by-step. Life changes are usually due to unexpected, chaotic events that create disruption and transition. Transitions are difficult and complex, yet they create opportunities for positive change. This newer, nonlinear model of psychotherapy is relationship-based in which therapist and patient(s) affect each other in an interpersonal, reciprocal relationship pattern. In psychotherapy, new self-organization may develop, leading to new thoughts and behaviors in relationships.

Couples like John and Maria influence each other constantly, in a minute-by-minute, nonlinear way. They establish patterns of communication—verbal and nonverbal—that are familiar and create the sense of knowing each other well. If these patterns become negative, entrenched, and repetitive, they create distance and hostility in the couple relationship. A helpful way of viewing these patterns is to conceptualize them as *fractal patterns* which constantly repeat.

Fractals (Tarlow, 2020) are never-ending patterns. They are infinitely complex patterns that are self-similar across different scales. They are created by repeating a simple process in an ongoing feedback loop, and create a larger pattern. When you look closely at the larger pattern, you can distill it down and discover the smaller pattern. Examples of fractals in nature are clouds, seashells, trees, flowers, and snowflakes. But fractals also exist in human behavior and show up in relationships. Couples often repeat the same pattern in an unrelenting negative cycle or until they reach a point when they are compelled to change.

Fractal theory is not the same as chaos theory. But chaos theory does have a place in fractal theory in that nonlinear dynamic systems exist on a spectrum ranging from equilibrium to chaos. A couple relationship system in static equilibrium does not have the internal dynamics to respond to the environment; as with other rigid systems, this response can cause the system to atrophy or cease to exist. Also, a couple relationship system in chaos has no viable pattern for communicating and stops functioning in a meaningful or predictable way. The most productive state to be in is "at the edge of chaos" where there is maximum variety and creativity, leading to new possibilities. In psychotherapy with couples, we aim to reach the edge of chaos in which the potential for change is maximized. Helping couples understand and recognize their self-repeating fractal patterns is essential for them to effect change.

Susan Johnson (Johnson, 2011), who developed Emotionally Focused Therapy for couples, describes these self-repeating fractal patterns in couple relationships as the "dance" and has identified common patterns as Pursuer-Withdraw, Withdraw-Withdraw, and Attack-Attack. John Gottman's (Gottman, 2013) method of couples therapy focuses on four destructive fractal patterns which undermine couple relationships: Criticism, Defensiveness, Stonewalling, and Contempt. In John and Maria's relationship, we find fractal patterns of Pursue-Withdraw and all four of Gottman's negative patterns.

As couples become aware of their fractal self-repeating patterns of behavior, they can experience these patterns in couples therapy sessions and work toward facilitating positive change together. Couples bring these fractal self-repeating patterns to each couples therapy session. The couple and their therapist become increasingly aware of their presence, both in and outside of couples therapy. Because fractal patterns are sensitive to initial conditions or small changes in patterning, therapeutic interventions—creating small changes in the way the couple experiences their fractal patterns—can create significant changes over time.

The interactive, nonlinear nature of couple relationships enables each member of the couple to be an agent of change in the relationship. Mary Main (1995) identified "earned secure attachment" made possible through the interactive secure patterns of change over a couple's history together. The network of minds in a couple relationship can generate new types of functioning that are fundamentally different from those in single minds. As mammals, we are social and not meant to go it alone. We are not meant to suffer separately. We need to feel and be with the presence of another, in order to bear what life brings us. We have seen this repeatedly during the pandemic where the effects of isolation have had horrific consequences throughout the world.

Individuals in couple relationships with "earned secure attachment" can begin to reflect on each other's experiences and form ideas about the other person's internal states, including feelings and needs. Fundamental attachment styles can be altered by couple dynamics to allow secure functioning together.

Fractal patterns may also exist within neuro-physiological responses such as the amygdala hijack which is an immediate, overwhelming, and out-of-proportion emotional response to an event which triggers a fight, flight, or freeze response in the amygdala. With John and Maria, an amygdala hijack response occurs when she discovers John's secret use of porn. Maria wants to both fight with John about this rupture in their sexual relationship, and to flee emotionally by withdrawing from John in a contemptuous way. The fractal nature of her response is clear in that an already established pattern of distrust in men was triggered by a self-similar event. In further revelations by Maria, we find out that her self-repeating pattern of distrust in men also contained her earlier sexual trauma: date rape when she was in her twenties. In sexual relationships Maria felt a strong self-repeating pattern of shame, self-blame, with fear of emotional and physical harm.

John also has a self-repeating fractal pattern of feeling worthless, unimportant, and unlovable. In their couples therapy, the therapist helps John become aware of these negative, embedded feelings and find words to describe them. He also begins to understand that he has patterns of flight and freeze when he feels worthless and unimportant. In therapy the "small change" of identifying and naming these negative and self-defeating feelings begins to create meaningful change and formation of new fractal patterns with more positive thoughts about himself. He begins to consider that Maria needs him and his presence, and that she values him as a person.

The therapist's calm persistence with John and Maria allows a complex interaction in their couples therapy which is neither rigid (allowing no change) nor wildly chaotic. The therapist becomes their temporary attachment person to guide them through the process of reflection and change. Indeed, their couples therapy can progress to a point in which there is a mixture of stability and variability that allows for gradual change. In this approach the therapist has time to learn and appreciate the couple dynamics, and the couple has time to process what they are learning together. New fractal patterns can gradually emerge, created by the non-linear and dynamic, thoughtful interactions between the therapist and the couple.

Another way to think about change in a couple involves complex "strange attractor" (Tarlow, 2020) patterns that capture the interplay between stability and change in the couple system. The couples therapist can serve as a strange attractor whose presence and interventions create new unfolding patterns in the couple's way of relating to each other.

Love itself involves strange attractors in each person as they are drawn to one another in hopes of creating patterns of stability through the unpredictability of life. In couples who view chaos or unpredictability in life as a barrier to avoid, they may try to maintain "sameness." However, periodic unpredictability allows for strange attractor patterns to emerge, leading to change and development. A couples therapist often serves as a "secure attachment" strange attractor, subtly influencing the couple's development of "earned" security with each other. The therapist's interventions within a secure base of treatment can guide the couple in modifying their patterns as they choose.

With John and Maria, the therapist identifies and moves energy from the familiar attractor point of their problems to the equally engaging strange attractor point. She creates a strange attractor pattern by guiding new emotional understanding of the couple relationship. She facilitates new meaning and challenges existing patterns. Maria says that the moment she is open and vulnerable, John turns away, while John sees Maria getting mad when he tries to engage with her. The therapist acts as a strange attractor with the goal of changing the pattern of distrust between them into a pattern of greater trust and security.

A couples therapist is also a strange attractor who influences couples with her own emotional state. Effective couples therapists maintain a sense of curiosity about each individual and the unique qualities of their couple relationship. Effective couples therapists also maintain hope for couples; they carry and convey hope for the couple's ability to change. The couples therapist's hope, curiosity, and interest are felt by the couple via their emotional brains (the limbic system). If the couples therapist creates a secure and safe emotional state in session, it allows the couple to risk change in well-established but negative fractal patterns. It is usually not *what* the couples therapist says (cortical communication) but *how* she shares her thoughts and nonverbally conveys her feelings with the couple (limbic communication). The limbic attractor connection draws couples together but may replicate a familiar, insecure, and dysfunctional familial relationship. The couples therapist, acting as a strange attractor, models and offers a different emotional experience to the couple. New ways of relating within couples therapy can also create a "butterfly effect" in which small changes can be the catalyst for larger changes in the couple relationship.

The concepts of fractal patterns, chaos theory, nonlinear dynamic systems, and strange attractors are helpful to understand what happens in couples therapy, and how new self and couple organization are facilitated. The couples therapist is essential in this dynamic unfolding of the couple relationship. Her ability to join the couple system "just enough" to understand them and carry hope is essential for positive and rewarding change.

CHAPTER 10

ZOOM AND EVERYTHING CHANGES
(SESSIONS 7 THROUGH 9)

It is noteworthy that this couple's treatment—in January, 2020—began in one of the most significantly challenging times in recent history. John and Maria came to my office with the expectation that we would meet on a regular weekly basis. There was nothing unusual about the scheduling. After entering the waiting room, we would sit face-to-face in the expected environment of my office, and then they'd leave through a privacy exit. They had a scheduled time, which was usually at the same time of the week. As they progressed, we'd meet after a workday, which made our sessions part of their winding-down activity. All of this was ordered, known, and predictable.

But then in March 2020, everything changed. As a nation, we were suddenly dealing with a crisis of the magnitude that had not occurred for over one hundred years. Suddenly, we were affected by a pandemic, an out-of-control disease that sent the terror of survival into all humans worldwide. There was absolutely no guarantee of safety for sure anywhere in the world. As a psychologist I will always remember the last day I was in my office, and I left without an idea that I would never return. But that is what happened. Overnight, we learned that we were all vulnerable to this microscopic danger that could overtake and kill us without notice. Fortunately, I have a home office, but I had no idea how to begin treatment and schedule on a platform called Zoom.

After we scheduled a time to meet, John and Maria—like my other patients—had to figure out how to talk to themselves and to me by looking into a camera. There was no more rushing to get to my office for a scheduled appointment. Was an appointment that occurred in the middle of the day easier because everybody was compelled to stay home? Perhaps, but we were in each other's space in a much different way.

Fortunately, my home office is separate from my house, so I did have some degree of having a sanctuary of my own. It is a short walk from my home to this outside unit, so both viscerally and internally, I feel a sense of privacy whenever I enter my space. But I became keenly aware that my clients might be affected because I am now in their personal space. Plus, since they can't leave their space/home, they are being affected by all that goes on around them. This has become yet another component of the couples work that I do.

This next phase of John and Maria's treatment no longer takes place in my formal office. This situation prompts me to "open the window" so you can see for yourself the challenge of having our sessions entirely online. What is quite apparent with John and Maria (as well as with many other couples) is their ability—in these brand-new conditions—to adjust to often-disruptive conditions. In one week, the normalcy of our world that was taken for granted was totally hijacked by this public health crisis. Doing couples work in the midst of this is a small sliver of a much larger picture of the conditions that are no longer under our control.

Just before our scheduled time to meet, I was more aware than ever of feeling concerned about the appointment with John and Maria. I had been doing Zoom sessions for about a week, and had already recognized the sense I had of being an intruder or voyeur into the patient's home. That meant "being in" their room, maybe even a bedroom, viewing personal possessions, and perhaps seeing how the couple lives that may be inconsistent with what I had previously known. For example, they may be more or less prosperous than had been acknowledged. And I could see who else might live in the house, how they interacted, and how the patient responded to inevitable interruptions from other phone calls or, in some cases, small children or other family members. These concerns were in addition to the constant concern of whether or not the technology will actually work.

> *I notice that they are sitting far apart, even though they are both visible on the screen. I immediately wonder (again) if they are in one of their cycles. They seem on edge, although I can't really be sure if I am reading the signs correctly. I am already feeling at a disadvantage because I can't read their faces in the same way that I can when they are in my office. But what is my option? We are in a pandemic, and this is the way it is going to be.*

Session 7

Dr. S: I am glad we could make this happen. I know it has been a big change for you. How are you each doing?

Maria: This situation is really devastating. It's bad enough that at my work I am afraid that they are going to terminate me because I am new to the team and have less job security than the other members. I just don't know how it is going to get better. The situation is so dire, and the news seems to get bleaker and bleaker each day. We're having enough instability, and this pandemic may just be the final blow.

Dr. S: I know you have been worried about your position there; this lockdown and having to work from home is really hard to manage. So, it makes sense that you are feeling more afraid. There are too many hurdles to climb all at once—a new country, a marriage, a new job, and now this. It's like you can't catch your breath.

Maria: Well, I can't. I am afraid most of the time even though John tells you how confident I am.

Dr. S: Of course, you are scared, Maria. It is hard on you to have so many changes to deal with at once. You have too many new roads to walk and navigate where nothing feels familiar or known.

Maria: (Looking more downcast and alone . . .) Well, I am alone. That's what I have been telling you all along, and I really can't do this anymore. I am sitting here saying this in front of John, and I already know that there is no point. He expects me to just deal with it and move on.

Dr. S: Maria, I hear your brain telling you what you can expect, and it seems as if it's urging you to not even try. What's the point? It sounds like you never thought that it was possible to actually say that you need help and support. Can you imagine doing this with John? Can you imagine turning to him, and letting him know that you really need him to be with you because of all that you are going through right now?

Maria: I have always imagined that someone in my life would help me this way, but I know that I've made it almost impossible to happen. I have kept my walls up so that I wouldn't need what I thought I'd never be able to get. I watched others get help, and I always felt sorry for them because they seemed spineless and weak. I promised myself that I'd never be in that position. I vowed that I'd rather be independent, even if it meant I was upset and worried much of the time.

Dr. S: So, you've made yourself be strong and even impenetrable because that's what you had to do, and how you had to cope. It's the way you have gotten through all kinds of situations and times that were hard for you. Am I understanding you and how you've felt underneath that armor? (As I am speaking to Maria and watching her on Zoom, I see her face darken; she turns away. I want to stay with Maria, but not overwhelm her when she is obviously moving into a more personal, emotional state.)

115

Dr. S: Maria, I can see from your face—from your eyes—that something is happening inside of you. Let's take the time to explore that.

Maria: I feel weird. I am getting really hot and uncomfortable sitting here. Part of me wants to get up and leave because I am not used to thinking about my feelings in this way. I don't let myself quit; I just keep going. But inside, deep down, all I have been feeling is relentless fear. I'm afraid of so many things, and I just thought that my only option was to put my head down and keep going. I had to keep it together.

> *I am watching John, and see him just sitting there. Is this too much for him? He has made it clear that he feels out of his league and uncomfortable with all of this emotional stuff. I want him to be there when she is opening up and softening. I don't, however, want this to backfire by engaging him before he is ready. Part of what I am trying to do is to expand each of their ability to stay with their feelings, but to do so in a more relational way.*

Dr. S: John, I know you're sitting near Maria, and looking into the camera. Can you turn to her, look at her face and her eyes, and tell me what you see?

John: (John turns toward Maria and he holds her in his gaze.) You really look sad and upset. I can see that your eyes are wet, and seeing you this way is hard for me. I know you've been talking about work and how tentative your position is, but I don't think

I realized how negatively this was affecting you. I just thought you were complaining about them not being fair to you.

Dr. S: So, you thought that Maria was just blaming the people she worked with because she felt they weren't acknowledging her situation and cutting her some slack.

John: Maria, if I really let myself go there, I know I was impatient because I heard your words as being dangerous to us. Every time you mentioned work it was like you were telling me that you weren't happy here. And when I heard those words, for me that meant that you were going to leave. Those two thoughts went together without me really thinking about you.

Dr. S: Oh, John, you're talking about your feelings of fear that come up inside you. Your brain is getting a signal that something dangerous is happening, and of course that makes sense because feeling that someone you love is going to leave is an awful experience.

> *All of this makes perfect sense because of John's lived experience of having a mother who basically abandoned him. He was with her when he was a small boy, but by the time he was into his teens she had descended into alcoholism and depression. This left a mark on his feelings of connection and consistency. Unfortunately, Maria's signals of fear and withdrawal are like arrows to his heart. It is hard for him to hold onto hope and perspective when he moves into this fear state.*

> 📖 *This is an example of Bowlby's internal working models that come alive in a relationship. John does not choose to go into this fear state. He does it without thinking because this is where his brain goes when he is in a fear-inducing situation. In an avoidant attachment style, fear of being abandoned is easily triggered with resulting emotional withdrawal.*

John: But sitting here I can see that you're upset because you felt that I did not understand, and I get that now. I get that you're frightened about losing your job, which has been the one stable and known experience that you've had since you came here. I guess I wasn't really thinking about you. I was just thinking about my needs, and your not being here. That felt awful and I didn't know how to talk with you about those feelings.

Dr. S: John, what are you feeling right now when you hear about Maria's fear, and that she is upset about now living in the US and the possibility of losing her job? What comes up for you?

John: Now that I am beginning to understand her feelings, which I really want to do, I feel bad and sad for her. And I want to make it better. I want to find a way to help her, and take on this rough situation together. It's not just her problem. I know that now, and I want to help her get through it because we're in this together.

Dr. S: John, you're feeling so much. Can you imagine saying this to Maria directly so that she can take it in?

> *I want this to be a felt and lived emotional experience. I know that Maria can "hear" his words, but we do not feel feelings from language alone. We experience our feelings in the moments and times when we feel our partner's actual lived efforts. I am "teaching" John to be with Maria by turning to her and speaking to her with his own feelings. That is what this prompt is all about. Some people need help and are uncomfortable with this. I imagine that John has had very little experience talking about his feelings, especially after being raised by an army dad and living on a military base. Sensitivity to each other's feelings is rare in that environment. I have to check with John to determine how he feels about this process.*

John: I feel like I just told her. I wanted her to hear that I do care.

> *A fear response again—a block—but hopefully it won't last or be too big.*

Dr. S: Of course. You did a good job, but I know you want her to understand that this is coming from you and you alone. It is just for her, and that's going to make a big difference for both of you. Does that make sense?

> *I am validating John's efforts because I know he has had little confidence in his ability to relate, and he is doing a good job of staying present in this uncomfortable, emotionally pulsing session. I want him to know and feel a sense of pride and accomplishment for*

> *his efforts in turning to his mate, so that this becomes an intentional relational experience. And as far as our hearts go, Maria will hear him differently when he speaks to her personally with his heart and just not his head. This will be more likely to happen when he is looking at her with his eyes.*

John: (Looking at her instead of the screen . . .) Maria, I feel bad that you have been carrying all of these thoughts that I was just pushing aside what you were going through. I didn't get how hard this was for you, and I can see that I was lost in my fear that you were going to leave, to give up on us. I know that I kept trying to tell you that you were making too big of a deal and to stop worrying about things. I can see now that you thought I didn't understand how much pain you are in. I should have never done that. I am so sorry for that and more.

Maria: (Pausing for a minute or so . . .) John, I want to believe that you mean this. I have been longing to hear those words for such a long time, and at least now you are trying. That means a lot to me. I can see that you're sitting here each week, and I know that this is hard for you. You told me that therapy wasn't something you have ever done, and that it's a white person's thing. So, it means a lot to me that you're making the effort now. I want you to know that, even though I can't stop thinking about what has happened in the past.

> *It's happening! Maria is starting to turn and become softer and more present. This is so important in terms of our work together. If she can allow herself to be more vulnerable and have needs, then it is possible for them to begin bonding and attaching. They need to do this because it is the foundation of having a more lasting relationship.*

Dr. S: (Watching Maria's face as she speaks . . .) Keep going, Maria. You are allowing this lovely moment to come. Let it in!

Maria: You're right. I feel the urge to say something negative, but I am learning to slow down that reaction. I do know that John is trying. (Turning to him . . .) I know you're trying, and that matters.

John: I thought I would never hear those words again. (As he speaks, he moves closer to her on the sofa and touches her hand.) I get that you need me, and I want to be here. I really do.

Dr. S: Go deep inside. Go inside and feel what happens when you start to close the fear and let your partner in. You're doing it now, so notice it. Your brain is always trying to protect you and you're making new connections, which actually begin to change the circuitry of your brain. These new neuronal connections will help you feel different in this relationship and in your life. This is important, and I want you to feel good about what you are doing together.

The Roller Coaster of Emotion

John: I feel kind of shaken about all of this. It's so new but I do want to be with Maria and most of all I want our love to grow. (As he says this his eyes are visibly moistened.)

Dr. S: It's a lot, John, and I see your feelings come alive. Can you let Maria see this? Can you turn to her so she can see your face? (John turns instead of looking at the screen.)

John: I do really want to be with you because I love you, I really do.

Maria: (Looking at John as he speaks . . .) It does make a difference when you look into my eyes. You used to do that when we first met and I didn't realize until just now how much that meant to me. I can feel your caring in such a different way. I am actually taking in that you feel bad about what has happened, what you said and did before.

> *I couldn't believe this happened on Zoom. It is such a challenge to work that way, and in this session, I was able to engage them in their actual emotional experience. That was difficult to do but they went there and it was definitely more than just a conversation. I am feeling that they are beginning to experience their connection as real. This emotional roller coaster seems to be evening out.*

Session 8

This is the first time that I am not feeling a sense of apprehension before my meeting with John and Maria. I noticed the palpable difference. The last session was not so contentious. I wonder if this will last or if it will change again.

And, of course, this perspective is based on my experience in couples work. Clearly, partners have bonding moments. But it takes many repeated experiences to interrupt and change established patterns. While John and Maria are not a long-partnered couple, their pattern of Withdraw-Withdraw has become a part of their highly defended relationship. I am looking forward to seeing them today, and only have mild reservations that come from not wanting to expect too much too soon.

I go to my Zoom account, send them the link, and within moments they are on the screen in front of me. Seeing them sitting closer, I am relieved that they seem more relaxed. This is definitely a good sign. At least the space does not feel as pulsating and intense as it had in the earlier session.

Dr. S: I have been waiting to see you and to explore what happened between you during our last session. Did that continue beyond the time we had together?

Maria: Well, it did for me. For the first time in a very long time, I felt easier with John and noticed that I was not having those constant thoughts of feeling alone and leaving. It wasn't like anything really changed, but I noticed that my mind just didn't go to that awful place. I remembered that you said I was having a fear response, and I think you're probably right. I never thought about it that way, but I have not felt able to trust John, and I think I was looking for signs that I was right. I can see now that has been like a trip wire that catches every move that you make. I know it's not right, but I couldn't stop myself from doing that.

John: I'm not glad to hear you say this, but I am somewhat relieved. I could feel it, and it made me upset because I felt like you didn't get what was happening—and that seemed even crazier. I had the same unsettled feelings of not belonging and being an outsider that I felt when I was younger. We moved around a lot to different bases because of my dad's job in the army. I had an awful time as a kid because I was always in between—I wasn't white and I wasn't black. I couldn't be part of the cool white kids' crowd, and I wasn't black enough to be accepted by the black guys who were jocks and tough, which I was not. I always felt that I couldn't get it right, and things got even worse when I was in my teens. Because of my skin tone, the other blacks called me uppity and pretty boy. I remember one of the black girls I tried to hang out with called me "conceited" when all I was doing was trying to have a conversation about some books that I was reading. I felt like a loser in the dating department.

When we first got together, I felt so special about you wanting me, but when you started pulling away it confirmed what I had feared all along. The message I got was that I was just not worth investing in, and that you didn't want me or any part of me. I felt this in my being, got angrier and angrier inside, and I know it came out against you.

Maria: I could feel that all the time, and I assumed that you didn't care about me anymore, which was further verified by the blame you kept heaping on me every single day. Why would I want to sleep with you and make love with you when all I felt over and over again was your anger and rage at me? I felt you had become my enemy, and who in the world sleeps with an enemy who is now trying to do you in?

> *Thankfully John and Maria are finally moving in the right direction. They are identifying the pattern that has kept them stuck in such uncomfortable feelings with each other. Those impressions are evoked because of their own lived experiences, which of course they carry in so many different ways. Their interactions began to cause fear and trepidation, even in relatively minor ways. It's like death by a million little cuts. It could be a misspoken word or a forgotten request. It could be something like being late when there was an agreement to be on time, or forgetting a date that was deemed to be important. These are ordinary moments that become painful, and are then seen as evidence of not caring. The case becomes bigger until there soon seems to be no turning back.*

Dr. S: Maria, you noticed that in the past you felt John's anger even though he didn't necessarily say anything about it.

Maria: That's really the problem because he never spoke to me, he never let me in. I just felt his anger. I could feel it in almost every interaction we had, and I wanted to know what was wrong. I really did. But when he didn't tell me what he was feeling, I concluded that I wasn't important. He didn't want to take the time and effort to talk to me, so I stopped engaging. I know I did that. I feel it must have really hurt you, John. I can see that now. And I am sorry for all of this. I never wanted to hurt you that way. I knew that once we came to the States it must have been hard for you, and that hurt me so much. I realized how many barriers there are for you as I heard and learned more about how Blacks are treated here. I was shocked because it is so different in my country, but I never said anything to you because I was afraid it would make things worse. So even though I was trying to protect you, I can see that you had no idea where I was emotionally or what I understood. That must have felt so isolating.

> *I am practically jumping up and down! This couple is beginning to work together and share their deepest fears and concerns. The hopelessness that seemed unending a couple of months ago is evaporating, and now there is only a small cloud instead of a dark horizon. When Maria lets John know that she feels pain for him, she is touching his deepest need, which is the same as for all of us—essentially, to feel our person is there and cares how we feel. When this does not happen, the world feels like an empty place—a bottomless pit with no place to go. I need to give them a perspective on this repetitive dance so that they can help each other when it begins to occur, rather than play it out over and over again.*

Dr. S: John, what is it like to hear Maria talk about how much she keeps inside herself because of her fear that she should not bring things up that might upset you?

John: I don't think she got there on her own. I'm sure I did my part to make that happen here as well. We've got to find a way to help each other so that that doesn't keep happening. I can see now that I've never known how to talk about feelings, and I probably made that pretty clear to her as well.

Dr. S: You're both owning what you have brought to the table, your own contribution of keeping the dance going. Making things explicit is a first and important step. But even more essential is being able to navigate the fear when it happens. I want to help you do that in the moment it happens, not just talk about it from afar.

Maria: I do feel empathy and concern, but I know that we have to talk about what has happened between us sexually and this is a conversation that never goes well. After today I feel hopeful about being able to talk about it here and we need to do that in order for me to feel safe and not want to turn around and go back home. I know I can't do that but that's my default mode when I feel that there is no understanding or concern for my situation.

Dr. S: Can you tell us more about what you are struggling with? You mentioned your concerns sexually, but please, let's hear more about what is going on inside you about all of this.

Maria: When we first met, John was really into me. We were like a couple of puppies, playing and fooling around all the time. I felt like this was our own special secret so that no matter what we were doing, I felt like I was his one and only. I remember this delicious feeling when we were out in the world. It was like I knew that I was different for him than anyone else in the world and that gave me a special sense of mattering and importance. But then we came to the States and life began to change. It was hard enough because for me everything was new and unknown. I kind of liked that for a bit but there really wasn't time for us. We had to move because John had been living with another friend. And then the whole immigration thing started.

If you want a killer for your psyche, deal with the US Department of Immigration. They treat you like you're an enemy trying to invade the country. Everything you do is suspect. I had a job with an international firm but that wasn't enough. We had to hire an attorney and then we decided to get married because at least it would give me the possibility of getting a green card. Without that I could not remain in the United States. I'm not used to feeling that I'm doing something wrong and that I am suspect of trying to pull something off. But that is the attitude of the immigration service.

And then my job began to get problematic. My skill set does not really go with the team that I've been put into. I'm concerned about that and I'm not sure what to do. And then I started noticing that John was on a lot of porn sites. I'm not exactly a prude but this was a deal breaker. I didn't feel like I could compete with those women, and besides, he seems to be drawn to that all the time.

John: Well, that is what happened because I was upset that you were so tired and always distracted. I felt like there was nothing between us after a while and that was pretty lousy. I saw this situation as the beginning of our end. And you know I did grow up in an army base and that was just what guys did. It was perfectly acceptable. In fact, if you were a full-blooded guy, that's what you did. I know I haven't been honest with you but I have been using porn since I was in my teens. It was one of the ways I felt normal. And then you came into my life and I wasn't that into it any more until we began to have our troubles.

Since I assumed that you didn't care, you were so absorbed in your own life, I didn't think it mattered. I know that I was wrong about this but I didn't know how to talk to you. And remember my father's words to me were always, "Don't expect anything from a woman. They tell you one thing and then they just do whatever they want." I figured you must have changed your mind and wanted someone who was more confident than me.

Dr. S: John, you are letting Maria see the parts of you that you've tried to hide and make disappear. That is a big deal. How are you feeling on the inside sitting here talking about these painful parts of you? You're taking this risk for the sake of your relationship and connection to Maria.

John: Part of me feels so weird saying this out loud. I can't believe I am sitting with you, a white woman, telling you about my porn use. It's hard enough with Maria and now there is you, a white therapist.

Dr. S: I can see that you are feeling this distress and I am grateful that you're telling me. What is it you think I am feeling now that I know this about you? Let's talk about that, because if we don't, it's going to sit here between us and take up space that will interfere with the work we are doing. Does that make sense?

John: Well, for starters I believe you must think I am some kind of pervert or creep. How could you not when I am talking about porn and we haven't even gotten into what I do which of course you know is to masturbate. I am certain that you think this is gross. And she does (looking at Maria).

> *There's that race piece again and of course it is going to be there. He's got reason to feel separate and different. I'm glad it is coming into our sessions, but I am always wondering if what I am saying and how I am as a person is really unbiased. I think I am an open person, but I know I have lived as a privileged person in a white world. I have had a protected, easier road to navigate in life. If I speak to him about how hard it has been for him, will I sound like I am placating him as if I could know what he has gone through? I do empathize with his feeling a sense of marginalization, because I have always cared deeply about belonging. But my wanting more is a white person's longings that come up when I am part of the system, not outside of it. I have come a long way since, in the past, I thought being color blind was the way to go. I am so concerned about my patient's differences; at times it really unsettles me. I am constantly reflecting on and expressing what I am feeling. I want to be sure that I am considering the patient and their inner world. The truth is that this sometimes feels exhausting and I do carry this in my body.*

Dr. S: John, you are one courageous guy. To risk letting me into your private place when everything about this is scary, and why wouldn't it be? I am sensing that the judgments you have encountered may also come up in our conversations. But those are not my feelings at all. I know that you've suffered the trauma of not fitting in and profound loneliness and you have coped by soothing yourself as best you could. That's what I am thinking and that makes me sad, very sad, for you and your suffering.

John: (Staring at me and Maria . . .) I am confused. This almost doesn't make sense. I have always believed I was one fucked up person and that was that. And what has been happening in my marriage has just brought this home. But now you are telling me you feel sad for me. That kind of sounds pathetic and makes me uncomfortable. But a tiny little piece of me way down inside feels something different. I have never said this out loud before but I have felt so unloved and awful I have wondered why I was here, why I was alive.

Dr. S: Of course, you have questioned your existence. When you have to travel through life alone, when you feel bad about the way you're trying to do it, at some point the emptiness becomes unlivable and unbearable. That is so understandable when you now have a partner. You longed for Maria to understand but she had no idea what was going on inside you. You figured that Maria wanted a different kind of man than you. (I look at Maria, who is again looking dejected and withdrawn.)

Maria: I am shocked. You're the one who lived here. You're the one with all the connections, not me. While I knew you had some feelings about where you came from, it never dawned on me to connect this to us. I feel bad about this, but part of me still blames you for not coming to me. Look what you've put us through because of your silence.

> *Maria's walls are hardening again. What is underneath this? What fear is driving her and causing her to move back into anger? Can I get her to put the armor down or is this too dangerous?*

Dr. S: Maria, I am noticing that wall come up again. What is happening inside? Can you slow down and touch that feeling that is deep inside you, that's causing you to become so prickly?

Maria: I keep seeing those images on his screen, you know the one's where they are having three-way sex and using all kinds of paraphernalia. I keep thinking that he's going to expect this from me and will never be satisfied with who I am and the way I function. It's terrifying to think that this is what my life is going to become.

Dr. S: You've become increasingly afraid. Can you imagine letting John know about this terror that is haunting you and filling your mind with very uncomfortable thoughts?

Maria: It's been so hard for me to even grasp what this all means. I feel his sadness and I hear where it comes from which is so sad for me to hear. But I am afraid that I am not able to be there in enough ways that he will need because I have my needs, too, and maybe we're both too broken to be with each other. I never knew that I could bring this up to him. I just began to conclude that we are different people and that he wanted a wife who is more open to sexual experimentation, which is not me. I need to sit with this and process what I am hearing today. I just need to feel that I am safe, and this is all happening so fast.

> *I find myself wondering how this session will end. Will they come in feeling closer and having a sense of hopefulness or will they continue to pull apart even though they had a few brief moments of repair during that last two sessions? Maria was beginning to soften and listen to John until he began to talk about using pornography to soothe himself after Maria left their bed. Obviously, this touched a raw nerve in Maria and she became reactive once more. Anyone who works with couples knows that the process is a slow one. We don't just surrender our beliefs which have been there for survival reasons. We have learned our own ways of being protective when we feel threatened, which is what happens when couples begin to pull apart. Couples therapy has to intercept these fixed beliefs and allow the partners to begin to consider another way of feeling. This is a big step especially when the external circumstances have been quite dire and challenging as with the actual loss of connection/abandonment that John and Maria mutually experienced. Knowing this, I am comfortable with the repeated process of Maria experiencing feelings of closeness and then moving into fear again.*

Session 9

The session began when I sent them the link for the Zoom appointment. Not having the initial and informal moments that were part of in-person sessions is a bit more challenging. Nothing is natural, such as when a couple walks from the waiting room into my office. The Zoom session begins and the couple is in front of you. I take a few moments to let them settle in and to gather a sense of where they are based on their body language and facial expressions. Sometimes I don't have to encourage them and create a space, because one or both will bring in something they are working on to talk about. This session began with silence which I did not want to interrupt, so for what seemed quite a prolonged time, no words were spoken. By temperament, I am a pursuer so my inclination is to dive right in, but I have come to appreciate how different our processes are and so I remained silent for the sake of the relationship and what each may be feeling. In this instance, Maria began to speak.

Maria: I left our session last week and was really upset again. I was able to calm down a bit when we were out of the session and I realized that my anger at John is my old way of trying to minimize something that I care about. If I make it unimportant and bad, then I don't have to care when something doesn't work out. And that's it. I am terrified, scared in my whole being, that our marriage isn't going to last. John has put me on a pedestal and seen me as impervious to fear and need. "You can do anything," he has told me, but inside, in the deepest recesses of my being, I am vulnerable and scared just like everyone else these days. There's this pandemic and having no control over our bodies and then there is my loneliness and feelings of loss about being away from the security of my family and country. I am not sure who I am anymore and all of this, on top of John turning to pornography, has been too much. My heart feels so much pain and constant sadness, I can hardly bear it at all. (As she says this, her eyes are moistened and almost closed.)

John: (He has been listening intently and when she finishes speaking, he does not miss a moment . . .) Speaking softly, he says, "Maria," and when she does not look up, he says her name more forcefully. I can't let this happen. I can't let you go into this dark, sad place feeling that I am giving up on you and us. I hear your pain and I can see how you could think I was more interested in the images on those sites, but that was just my effort to numb myself into not feeling because I was becoming overwhelmed with my longings and desire for you. Please hear me. I hear you like I have never heard you before and I want to make sure you know that. Please, Maria, try to open your heart to me. I love you and I am so sorry that I was not there when you needed me. You have had to make so many, many changes and I know I felt guilty that you had to do this and not me. I kept berating myself feeling that I was not being a strong and real man because you were carrying a heavy, heavy load. I know I never told you this but I felt this so many times. I wish I could have known how to share this with you because now it seems so easy.

The Roller Coaster of Emotion

> *Will his efforts to reach her be successful? Can he penetrate the armored coat that she wears because of her constant sense of potential danger and loss? I need to be quiet and patient and let her feel her feelings herself. The last thing she needs is to feel pushed. Of course, that would cause her to become more walled off and reactive again.*

Maria: (Looking at John for a few long minutes . . .) You really do want me, don't you? I can hear in your voice, and I know you pretty well now, that you really mean this. And I find myself wanting to hear more and to believe you. Maybe it is your energy and voice, you really do sound intense and that matters to me. I want to feel wanted, really wanted, because that makes a huge difference to me. I feel like you're fighting for me. Usually, I feel that I am just taken for granted, a function, someone who just is supposed to do whatever needs to be done. And when I feel that way, you have seen me. I become angry, resentful, and attacking and when I am worn out, I give up and go away. I am sorry for that. I know I can be a mean, ungiving person and that's not the me I want to be with you.

John: I never wanted to come to this couples therapy, but I am so glad that we got here. I am sorry that I fought you on this as well. It's like we were living in the basement and I feel like I am in the light and upstairs for the first time in a long time. I can see how I missed the signals you were sending and I am committed to working on this for as long as it takes. What I keep hearing in my heart is that you want to be my wife again. You want to stay with me.

Maria: You're right about that and even more. I want to learn and help you with those painful feelings from your lonely childhood because I care that you have suffered. We both have suffered and we've got to help and change that by being with each other in a supportive and healthy way.

I can see that because that's what you did today by coming toward me, by insisting that you wanted me even though I was turned away and blocking you in every way possible. But you didn't let me keep doing that. All I have ever wanted was for someone to want me enough that when I am frightened and going into my painful fear in anger and rage, they would still care and want to help me. It feels so different and I can stay here now. I want to stay here now. I really, really do.

> *This is one of those times that I feel satisfied as the therapist. That does not happen too often. With all the traumas that this couple has had, they are moving in the right direction of being able to be with each other in a different way. They really do have a connection that is greater than just the original physical attraction. They have lots of work to do, but they are beginning to do what they need to do to build their foundation. They are each expressing their understanding of what they are bringing to this relationship. That is essential in order to recognize that it is a shared relational problem rather than being a blame game between them.*

Chapter 11

The Path Taken

There have been a number of sessions since you first met John and Maria. They have had to deal with the major issues that began when their relationship changed from a playful engagement to a more serious commitment. Of course, this makes sense since the playfulness of their early relationship was about attraction driven by the biological imperative to mate and reproduce. This is part of the evolutionary push to keep our species as mammals alive and thriving. The oxytocin and adrenaline in our brains cause us to become immediately and magnetically engaged. Our brains are taken over by an excited state and, even as humans, we are not in the mind-set to think about the consequences. This is the basis of the expression "madly in love" or infatuated. This is biologically imperative for all mammals, big and small. We can't fault John and Maria for what they could not do or understand. They were just being mammals.

Initial Attraction

Initial attraction to a partner involves physical attraction, ease in conversing, emotional attraction, optimum shared values, and similarity.

An important aspect of initial attraction is mood: does the person create a good mood for us and vice versa. John was initially attracted to Maria because she laughed, joked, and created a good mood for her friends and later for him.

Initial attraction also involves being playful with each other and putting each other at ease.

But then they found themselves in real life. Maria left her family and ease of life behind with the hope and very real expectation that her personal commitment to do well would give her a way to succeed in both her relationship and her profession. While John and Maria are well-intentioned people, they each had their issues from their own lived experiences. This translated into the way they felt about themselves and about others. They attempted to navigate these normal challenges of their new relationship but in addition—not that they could have predicted this—they also came together at a time of cataclysmic change and chaos: in politics, climate, and in health, with the deadly COVID-19. Anxiety and fear, not calmness, became the condition for many individuals and therefore many couples. Bruce Feiler (2020) coined the term "life quake" to describe such evocative events during which the individual experiences himself un-moored, his foundation shaken to the core. He posits that at the time of a life quake, humans often make major changes in the direction of their life. So, it makes sense that the convergence of these experiences left John and Maria off kilter, highly unsettled, stumbling in their lives, and

> *feeling ill-equipped to manage this alone. The good news was that even in this heightened dysfunctional state, they knew enough to seek out the help of another, the couples therapist. Perhaps as you remember the first few sessions, there may be more sensitivity to what each of them was going through. They were truly experiencing a life quake based on the internal experience that neither felt the other was there in a supportive and meaningful way.*

The sessions that came after the first few months continued to deal with the themes that emerged at the beginning of therapy. Each began learning and understanding more about the other's pain. They learned that their individual pain was the result of feeling fear and aloneness. They had their own way of trying to signal the other about their internal experience and their painful emotional state.

Maria was going through a difficult time realizing that her job and the success that she had previously taken for granted were no longer as certain now that she was a foreigner living in a new country. In America, even with her skills and personality, she was at the bottom of the hierarchy and was not feeling secure in her work. In Italy, she had a large network of friends she enjoyed and who supported her in the various changes that she made. This support was quite different when she came to live in America. She no longer had easy access to long-standing friends which was a difficult and painful change to manage. She also had to navigate the unending maze related to immigration issues made even more difficult because of the administrative polices that were in place. Maria always believed that America was the land where one could immigrate and realize dreams by working hard and being productive. Between the gates of immigration that had grown high and were difficult to open, and a job where her previous accomplishments were essentially not valued, she began to question if she were where she needed to be. Trying to communicate this insecurity created much distress because John saw her pessimism and anger as a sign that she was giving up on their relationship. As he pushed her to be more sexual, she felt even less understood and more upset. Their bonding became conflictual and angry. They pulled further and further apart.

With the COVID-19 pandemic raging throughout the country, everyone, no matter how secure they had previously been, felt bombarded by the uncertainty of the epidemic's force that was sickening many in its path. John and Maria no longer had their usual social outlets that had provided balance and perspective. They were confined to the four walls of their home, as was everyone. The timing of this was quite detrimental as they had just begun to build their social and personal lives together here in the States. While their small one-bedroom apartment was attractive and modern, it was not laid out in a way that gave them each a private workspace that would be more conducive for their jobs. In effect, their home became a prison that they could not leave. This made the initial phase of their new marriage even more difficult.

And then their own unresolved issues, from their feelings about themselves and their previous lived experiences, began to take over. Neither felt loved, cared for, understood, or considered. It was like each of them was living on their own island being buffeted by the waves of life. Neither felt the other was interested or cared about what was happening, so trust and safety came into question.

The middle sessions of therapy dealt with these emerging issues as they came up in the events of everyday life. John let Maria know more about his sense of being a biracial man in a country where he regularly felt he had to prove himself and was never sure if he was good enough. He let her know that this was what he feared, this was what he felt when he believed that she, like others who had come before her, was not satisfied with him. Maria had not fully grasped the extent of this kind of marginalization that was part of John's experience.

An example of this occurred when he was up for a review in his job. There was a lot of instability in his company because of the pandemic. John came into the session very upset because one of his close friends had just been given notice.

Dr. S: John, you are watching this happen and it's like you are seeing the cracks in the ship and wondering if it is going to go down with you on the deck unprotected.

John: It's that and more. Maybe you two white women can't imagine this, but I have learned to always be watching my back. No matter what, as a non-white person, I know that if there are cuts being made, I can't be sure that I'll be protected. In fact, my experience tells me that I won't. I don't have the same connections in my industry as people have where their parents have positions in their communities. They've belonged to the right groups. They are known. I've had to work and make my place and in times like this, who you know counts. I don't have any of these protections and I never have. And right now, I fear more than ever that I never will.

Dr. S: I can hear how hard this is for you. You have worked so hard and sometimes there are barriers that have prevented you from getting to where you have wanted to go. It's that privilege thing again, right?

John: Do you really understand this? I am never sure that any white person can. I try not to let it take over me but it's there all the time even if I try to keep it out. It's what I learned, what I was told, ever since I was a little kid. When Maria and I got together, I thought it would be over. But that was my mind playing tricks on me. Not only is it not over, it is even bigger in some ways. You should see how some white guys look at me. I can see their hatred, their anger at me for being with her and that's in there, too. And I didn't want to tell her. I thought I should just manage it myself. You have no idea how torn up I am.

Dr. S: You mean you thought you should just keep it to yourself and deal with these feelings as something that was part of being a husband, part of being a mate.

John: Well, you're right about that. I'm learning in here that I need to talk about what's going on inside of me, but it's really difficult when my whole upbringing had to do with being a strong, impenetrable person who knew what they wanted. I've been faking that for so long, it's hard to do otherwise.

Maria: John, I know that I am only beginning to really understand how you have suffered. Hearing your fears and how you have tried to protect me makes me feel sad, so sad that we've been so separate. I can see how that has created even more damage when there was already plenty of hurt in that area. I want to be there and I want to be the person that you come to. I want to know what has happened and why you are upset. Please, please don't protect me. It only makes things worse because I can feel your distance and then I feel like I don't matter.

Dr. S: Maria, I am listening to you and how John's feelings are coming into to you. And I am noticing John sitting there and wondering what is going on inside of him. Can you tell Maria what it was like to hear her say this, to hear her wanting to be there for you?

John: I heard her for sure and the words are so nice but I know there's a part of me that is still afraid this is just for this moment. I want to believe you really are here with me but part of me can't quite believe that it will last, that you won't change your mind, especially if I mess up in any way again.

Dr. S: I am hearing your fear coming up again like a herd of wild horses, rushing into to you and taking over. Your brain is trying to protect you from being hurt again even while your heart wants to open and take her in. Can you even imagine telling her this, telling her how you need her reassurance about being there and not threatening to leave because it causes you so much pain, the kind of searing, life-sucking pain that takes over?

John: (He turns to Maria . . .) I hear what you are saying but I need your help in letting me know that you want me to be safe and trusting. I need you to remind me that you really care and don't want me to suffer. I can't believe I am saying this, but I need you, Maria. I need you to want me and to let me know, because believing I am wanted is difficult and I end up feeling crazy and unlovable.

Maria: (Her eyes are fixated on John and without a word she reaches over to hug and touch him and begins to cry.) I am so sad and sorry for what has happened. I feel how awful this has been for you and I want to make it better, for you and for us. I can see my part in things and I want to change all that. I never knew I was important enough to anyone and I can see how wrong I was. I want to work with you on this and I commit to doing my part to change the anger that I have unleashed on you.

John: I can feel that you're with me. It's amazing. I never believed I'd feel this way with anyone, especially a woman. I just want to sit here with you so that this moment will keep going on. This is good, Maria, really good.

Maria: I am here, John, and I know where I need to be. I want you to feel the goodness about yourself and us. You are a good person and I am here to stay.

> *Feeling tears in my eyes, which I was fine for them to see, this was a true time of bonding that we all felt together. I didn't want to enter their special moment and told them to be with each other and not look at the Zoom screen at all.*

THE PATH TAKEN

This session marked a turning point in John and Maria's journey. The change inside of each of these good people began to occur after this session as they each courageously allowed their fears to come into the light of day, to be spoken about and seen with their partner as witness. These real moments were fundamentally different than what each believed would be possible. These bonding moments marked this couple's journey in earning a more secure relationship based on commitment and lasting love. Our hearts don't change unless we feel the true presence of another person who is tuning into us, unless we feel the effort to support and to really try to understand what is going on inside our hearts. That is one of the reasons why the repetitiveness of treatment is so essential. This relearning of our brains takes many repeated experiences over time. That is how we literally build new neuronal connections.

Neuroplasticity (Cozolino, 2006) is the overall process through which our experiences alter our brain connections. This process allows us to learn anew—to change our thoughts and our feelings. Fortunately, our brains are capable of change throughout our life span.

Many of us are born into situations that are challenging and even detrimental, often referred to as the birth lottery. Obviously a child does not pick the circumstances into which it is born. Lucky is the child who is cherished and cared for, lives in home that is sufficiently protective, and has enough to eat on a daily basis.

But the majority of the world lives with conditions that are quite different: harsh environments, scarcity of food and shelter, and often serious political and social unrest. Added to this are individuals who experience specific traumatic events such as loss from sudden death, illness in the family, an accident involving a close family member, or even changes in the family structure due to any of these traumas.

These losses and changes are hard on the human nervous system, and often cause disruption to healthy functioning throughout the individual's lifetime. These individuals often suffer from worry and fear that affects how they engage with their own offspring and other family members. Does this mean they will be burdened with this very real anxiety forever? Is there any way they can find a more secure existence after the frights that have been part of their lives?

The brain is basically a plastic structure that can change. We can alter our bodies medically by taking a pill, changing our diet, or undergoing an operation. But we have to deal with our emotional difficulties differently. For people who have suffered from trauma and loss, the circuitry of their brains is bathed in fear-inducing experiences that cause the circuitry to become extremely reactive and easily triggered. The brain learns this fear responsivity because of our social nature; it is through the same circuitry that we need to make our changes so that the relationship then becomes the instrument of the healing.

As we mature, these patterns of behavior continue to take place in our relationships. But it is possible to heal these earlier ruptures by consciously forming social relationships that are more supportive and trusting. One of the purposes in writing this book is to emphasize the conscious aspect that we believe is essential to directly effecting the healing process.

Some adults are able to successfully form more caring relationships and engage with others to "earn" the security that was so elusive when they were younger. Many of us, though, continue to repeat the same patterns of relating that duplicates the anxiety and reactivity of our earlier experiences. Therapy—couples or individual—is structured to examine these patterns and work through them with the help of the therapist, who becomes part of the healing process. The dynamics of the process activate the attachment circuitry that can be worked with in a caring and careful way. The therapist, understanding the attachment wounds that have occurred, pays attention and works with the arousal problems that have plagued the person. To quote Louis Cozolino, a psychologist who studies emotional processing, "The activation of both affective and cognitive circuits allows frontal systems to reassociate and reregulate the various neuronal circuits that organize thinking and feeling" (2002, p.308). When this occurs, unlike when the individual was younger and overtaken by the awfulness of the experience, they now learn to think and have language so they can stay in the moment and feel the experience that had been so elusive.

But this relearning is a messy business. The therapist has to be in the dysregulation, in the pain, and somehow maintain their footing. There is no one method on how to do this. The limbic system was overtaken originally; the revision does not occur by words alone and certainly not in a single moment. This is the complex basis of brain changes that are possible over time.

Dr. S: So much is happening here today and clearly you are beginning to be with each other in a very different way. This change is helping you create a foundation. It is literally changing the pathways of your brains.

Maria: (Her face darkens again . . .) You are talking about our brains. I want to share something that is happening right now, right this moment. It's like I feel close to John but at the same time I find myself going back to his using pornography. What's wrong with me? I feel bad about this thought but I better let you know this because I don't want it to take over as it has in the past when I find myself remembering what he did. I don't like that I go there so I thought I should bring this worry in here because I know you'll help us with this big thought and fear that I can't contain.

Dr. S: Maria, I am so glad that you feel safe enough now to know that you can bring something up so we can process it together. I want to note that this is a big change for you.

Unlike the earlier sessions of blame and shame, Maria explained that she wanted to understand what this was about because she felt she had a part in what had happened. She began to reflect on her experience growing up in a Catholic world. While she was no longer religiously oriented, she noted that she still carried a more traditional perspective. Coming of age in a female-dominated household, Maria's experience was to view sex from that mind-set. She realized that she did not have brothers who looked at porn, and that her mother viewed porn as something that only weird people engaged in. Seeing her husband stimulated this way added another nail into her heart that was already feeling quite uncomfortable. For Maria, this meant that he was no longer interested in her, that he had found something that was more fun. She even remembered her mother warning her, "If your husband starts to look at other women, you can be sure he is ready to move on. Don't kid yourself, that's just what men do. They never stay put." You can imagine the older women of her culture had overt disdain for any sexual interest outside the sanctity of the marriage. Maria stated that she did not even know how to talk about this. She actually had no language.

Here is a look at how this played out in other sessions that followed.

Maria: I still have to bring this up. I can't stop seeing you in front of that screen and every time I want to put it out of my mind, those images of you sitting and masturbating are still there. (As she is speaking, her voice gets quieter and quieter.)

Dr. S: Maria, your voice is barely audible. It's like you're having a hard time speaking.

Maria: I don't know what to say. I was never supposed to think about that kind of behavior. I knew that my mother would be horrified. I was supposed to be a good and proper girl. I heard her and my aunt talk about girls who were otherwise and I knew early on that I could not ever let anyone think that I was into anything involving sex. I wasn't supposed to be interested in that at all. Not ever. But I was interested in sex and sensual things. I watched movies and saw the popular singers. I knew they were different from my mother and my aunt. I wanted what I thought they had . . . freedom to be in the world. But then things got confusing. After I went to university and had that awful shaming experience, that man violating me, I felt such profound shame . . . unbearable feelings of badness . . .

I wasn't sure what was all right with sex. Meeting John seemed like the perfect solution. I felt that I could keep my secret because we came from such different places. He would have no way of knowing anyone who knew me so there would be no reason for him to know. I needed that anonymity to feel safe and comfortable in getting to know him sexually. There was no one to see or know or ask questions. I was protected, or so I wanted to believe.

And it was fun and wonderful. It was like we were in our own world. And then it just stopped. We came to the States and all we have had is one problem after another. The worst has been my terror about work. I was so upset with myself that I was not creating a place where others wanted to work with me, where I was valuable. I have never felt this kind of shame about who I am. I would come home and all I wanted to do was to tell John how upset I was and disappointed with myself because I felt like a loser. I wanted him to hold and comfort me, and instead all he did was question me about what I could do to try harder.

That did it. I felt even more alone and unseen. And John was right when he said I gave up on him. I was hurt and angry and I wanted to punish him so I shut myself away and stopped trying to talk to him. I kept asking myself what kind of person I was for having those feelings. I felt like I was a bad, crazy lady so I just shut myself off assuming that that was what he wanted, too. I felt I had to go, leave and not come back.

John is looking at Maria as she speaks and his gaze is visibly sharpened as she describes her pain. Without a prompt of any kind John moves closer and touches Maria.

John: I guess I never fully realized the depth of your suffering and pain. I did feel your anger and it felt like the love was gone. And I know that I, too, felt crazy, alone with your going away, your back to me, as if our relationship didn't matter at all. The most awful part was that I felt like I couldn't stop you. I felt impotent in every way.

Dr. S: Do you hear the word you are using? The word impotent. Let's really appreciate your word.

John: Impotent. When you make me pay attention to myself, I can see why I went back to porn and self-satisfying myself. It was my way to keep my manhood. And it was just that. At least for a bit of time I felt my manhood. It's what I learned to do growing up; it's what all the guys I knew did. And then when you saw it and said the things you said, I felt that the last nail had been placed in the coffin in terms of our relationship.

Maria: Oh, John, I am so sorry I made you feel so bad about something that is so basic. I realize now that my view of what is our right about our bodies was based on the way I was raised which was really constricted. I thought I was done with that provincial way, but I see that I've carried this into our relationship and I feel really bad about that. I see that in some way my attack on you was actually an attack on myself and my own version of self-hatred and disgust.

John: Maria, it hurts me to my core to hear the pain you've been in. I wish I had known how to be with you when you were suffering. I found you so attractive and sophisticated that I assumed you were really sure of yourself and that you could handle anything that came your way. In our relationship, I could tell that I had more need for actual sex than you and again I assumed that was just a guy thing. What do I know about this? They make you go to school for so many things but no one ever helped me understand about my own drives and needs. I kept that to myself just like I did about everything that goes on inside me. It was too risky to do otherwise.

I guess eventually, because you matter so much, keeping these feelings inside has become more and more difficult. I needed and wanted you while at the same time you were shutting down and going more into yourself because of how upset you were about what was happening in your life with me and in the job that used to be your place of accomplishment and success. I didn't know what to do with your disinterest.

I tried to tell you, which failed because I now know I was a jerk in the way I did it, going at you, berating you, telling you what a bad wife you were being. I can't believe my stupidity. What was I thinking? I just was trying to get you to see how upset I was. And when you went even further away, that's when I began watching porn again. The truth is I used to watch it quite a lot, especially when I was upset about anything. It was a relief to have that way to take care of myself. Please, Maria, try to understand that I am not blaming you, but please see that it was something that happened between us. I know now that we both have been in a lot of pain.

I appreciate that you are looking at your part of this and I feel so much better now that we can talk about what is going on.

Dr. S: John, can you imagine turning to Maria with your feelings right here, right now? Can you let her see your face as you tell her what you are experiencing inside, in your heart?

(As I said this, John stops looking at the screen, faces Maria, and looks into her eyes. I wish we were in person, but Zoom is what we have.)

John: No more blame. I know I have a part in this and I just want us to be with each other. I want to be part of your feeling more comfortable with your body and mine. We can do it, I just know it, I do. I really know now what my watching porn has meant to you and I am so sorry for all of this and more.

Maria: (She looks at him for a few minutes.) I can really feel you are not blaming me. I know that I've had that wall up for the longest time because I kept feeling that you were disappointed in me. Maybe that comes from the way I was raised. There were so many expectations that it was difficult to feel satisfaction and success. You know the term "good enough" has no meaning for me. It is either you're perfect or you've failed. When I heard and read in your eyes that you wanted more from me, I immediately felt like I was not good enough and all my wild childhood fears came alive inside of me. I wanted to talk with you about all of this but I had no idea how to do that and felt even more shame for having this need. It just felt worse and worse.

Dr. S: Look at what you're able to do and how are you talking to each other. I am sitting here watching you listen and be with each other in a kind and considerate way. Pay attention to how you are feeling this in your body, how you feel this in your being. What do you notice? Is it different from before?

John: I do feel relaxed. I can't believe I'm sitting here talking about my own self and my feelings. And it doesn't feel so weird anymore. I used to think of myself as an island, impervious to anything else. I don't want that anymore. I want to just be here with you, Maria, and to learn how to we can help each other and stop this pattern of blaming that we have engaged in.

Maria: (She sits there quietly, so different from before.) I am actually hearing you and I don't have that anger thing coming up as I have in the past. I heard your effort to understand where I have been and not blame me as I have felt in the past. And I am looking at you through my eyes that feel the loving that I used to see and I am feeling now. It feels so different. I can feel that you want me and because of that I want to tell you and talk to you and have your help with this mess that I get overtaken by. I believe once more it's us against that bad world. You're my man! (John is beaming.)

> *When a couple makes this kind of turn, I feel such a sense of pleasure and joy. It moves me to the core, even to the point of tears. I can't fake that. It is what happens when I am really touched as they open their hearts to each other. It truly is a magical moment. I want to savor it with them, and I do. At the same time, I know that while there is more work to be done, I have to nurture their confidence in being able to maintain this connection on their own. Does this sound parental? Maybe it is, but in attachment terms I know I am the temporary attachment figure that has stood by and helped them recognize their own power to make the changes that will increase their relational experience. Can every couple do this? Of course not. But if the partners commit to the process of learning about each other, more often than not, the caring increases.*

Dr. S: I am appreciating the gains you have made in risking that turning back, in needing each other, and silencing that old brain's efforts to keep you safe—to keep you connected to the past and the dangers you encountered. But you took that risk in session today and you have done it before. Importantly, you're noticing the difference and celebrating it together. I look forward to hearing more about it when we meet again.

Because couples in intimate relationships are emotionally attached, they are continuously affected by each other's feelings and emotional states.

This primary partnership is unlike that with any other human being. With a friend, even a close one, you may feel disappointment or some sadness, but because you are not primarily attached to that person, those feelings usually do not interfere with the relationship. But it is different with your primary person, your mate, the person you have entrusted your heart with. If things are going well, you may have noticed that your life feels all right. If you are having relational problems, life may seem unmanageable, even unlivable. Relational distress is like being in a dark ocean with no shore or light in sight.

The term disruption refers to the states that occur when one or both partners are triggered and become aroused. Relational conflict may result from tiny breeches: forgetting to call, coming home late, being dismissive in some conversation, falling asleep when the other is talking, not listening to the partner's words, and working on a project rather than going to an activity. Each of these experiences in and of itself is likely not of major importance. But if there is an accumulation of incidents where there is a lack of presence or concern, they become important and may cause relational conflict. It is as if the partner begins to feel, "I cannot depend on you." This becomes even more problematic if there is a breech in trust from major injuries such as in infidelity and emotional abandonment or not being there during a time of need or transition. These painful experiences cause a disruption in the attachment bond which reverberates in the couple relationship. It is as if there is actually a block or barrier between the partners. If the injury is not dealt with, each partner continues to feel unsafe, uncared for, and begins to emotionally withdraw from the relationship.

The attachment relationship is a living entity. In order to survive when there is a disruption in this bond, both partners have to commit to the process of looking at what has caused the disruption. This is not a simple process since each partner has their own feelings and beliefs about themselves and their partner. It is often difficult for partners to feel safe enough to reveal the hurts and pain they carry about the experience that has had such meaning. Doing this is especially problematic for individuals who have not felt understood or cared for in earlier attachment relationships. Their brains remain locked in fear—for good reason—because trusting was not a learned experience.

Repair is not an illusion and something only a few couples can achieve. Repair comes from the hard work of prioritizing the relationship. This means committing to reflecting on one's own feelings and the behaviors that result when the fears come alive in the relationship.

This was what you saw as you went through the narrative with John and Maria. Their attachment began in an idealized way, but started to unravel as they each became overtaken by their fears and feelings of insecurity both from the present and previous relationships. In the treatment, they began their commitment to being with each other and to turning back to try to listen to each other's pain, as challenging as it was. The injuries had to be acknowledged and grieved and recognized for what they had caused. This repair becomes part of the couple's new lived experience and hopefully leads to a more secure emotional connection that can weather the future challenges that will arise.

Our Last Few Sessions

Maria: I know things aren't perfect, but I actually feel like I can breathe, like things are going to probably be okay. I can see how we got to where we did and while I know we have a lot of work to do, that feels completely normal just like you say to us all the time. I like the idea that we have to work at building our relationship. You've given us the courage to feel that that is possible. That's such a different perspective than when we first started coming to see you. It feels like a lifetime ago even though it was only about a year ago when first began to see you. Did we tell you what we do on the weeks we don't see you? (They exchange a look with each other.)

John: Your name is our cue. When we start getting into the "weeds," that word you have used so often, then one or the other says, "Dr. S," and we both know what that means. It reminds us that we are amping up and we know that is dangerous and will not be productive.

Maria: That's what is happening now and we both feel good about how we are being with each other. We were wondering if it makes sense for us to come less often. We want to try to do this on our own. You've given us the tools and we want to be our own resource, just like you told us early on.

John: We hope you understand that this is about us and not a sign that you're doing something we don't like.

Dr. S: It means a lot that you are bringing your thoughts into this session about stopping your therapy. Because I'm hearing this from both of you, I appreciate that it is a mutual decision. Well, I am glad that we can discuss this decision because I want to talk about what you have done so far and consider what matters you may still want to pay attention to.

Maria: Does this mean you feel that we are doing something too quickly or that we are being foolish about this decision?

Dr. S: I am appreciative that you're asking this and it gives me an opportunity to be with you in the fullest way possible. I support your growth and confidence in wanting to be on your own. What I want is for you to have a road map that you can refer to regarding the important things you are working on in this building process. Does that make sense? Can you hear that as me supporting your own maturation and learning process as a couple?

John: We have learned so much about ourselves and I know we've got to keep focusing on this. We have been so much better about recognizing our raw spots and how these come up at times and take over. I know I have to work on going into my insecurities the minute something interrupts our easy relationship. I carry a lot of baggage as man of color.

> *This is the moment that all therapists have to manage, or at least those of us who work and become attached to our patients. It is not a question that I want them to stay indefinitely, because this personal effort to move on, mutually expressed, is quite meaningful. But on a purely personal level, it is a loss. While I know it is essential, this still changes the pattern of our work and connection. I do not need dependency, but in the best possible scenario, couples like John and Maria keep in touch intermittently. My experience is that that is beneficial for them and for me. Connection is like that and the last thing I want to*

> *do is to make this a business transaction that ends with the door closed once and for all.*
>
> *Over the years I have come to understand that every person is different about their relationship with me and the work we have done together. The real payment, at the deepest level, is when couples and the individuals whom I have seen continue to maintain a relationship with me in some way. That may mean an occasional call or email, or for some it is a card at Christmastime. All of this speaks to the connection that we have made, and I am honored to become part of their attachment system. As we explained at the beginning of this book, attachments are about the connections that give meaning and purpose to our lives. John and Maria found their way back to each other and began to work on building their relationship through caring and attention. Hopefully they will continue this work and effort even though they are no longer in therapy.*

Maria: And I know that I have to mind my escalation and withdrawal which can cause me to become cold and unresponsive. I have to work on recognizing when I am moving into this quickly and slow this down, get off the road, and give myself time to calm down and get back to my mind instead of just reacting as if John is my mortal enemy. My Buddhist friend calls this staying in my seat. I can see now how important this is if I am going to be the loving partner that I long to be. It means a lot to me that you think I can do this.

Dr. S: What I hear is your mutual vulnerability in now being able to let each other know how important you are to each other, and to let each other know about the deeply meaningful commitment and attention you want to make to support this relationship. Look what you have been able to do when you allow yourselves to be close and connected to your heart and your longings, when you take down those walls and armor. I look forward to hearing that you are continuing to work on this. You've come together in our work to begin creating that secure base. I want to make sure you know that even though you will not be coming in for appointments regularly, I am here and will continue to be as we have a relationship together that is there for you to use in the future. Living in a relationship is work. This is the same for all of us as humans living in a complex and uncertain world. Please remember that you can open the door again at any time you want to work on some situation or process issues that feel a bit tangled.

The therapeutic experience is about creating a secure base from which the couple can develop a sense of earned security together. Once greater security is established in the process of couples therapy, the couple can experience increased safety and trust with each other. Regular therapy is no longer essential to their well-being but the therapist continues to serve as a secure attachment figure they can return to if needed.

> *If you are thinking that I am validating their process and experience, you are correct. I do this intentionally because this effort to stand on their own feet is part of the therapeutic process. It is what makes therapy a corrective experience. Many people long for support from the important people in their lives, but sadly for many, such as Maria and John, that did not happen automatically. Knowing this, I hope to create a different process of engagement and collaboration. This conveys the basis of any relationship: I respect you and support your efforts to be there for yourself. I do want to convey this belief in the way I engage with couples, including when they are deciding to step out of regular contact with me. Like learning to swim in deep waters, the dip into this therapeutic experience does not just last for the moments we have met. The aftermath hopefully continues and with a process of curiosity and reflection now more permanently in place.*

Chapter 12

In Conclusion

We wrote this story about a young, newly connected couple but want this book to be relevant to partners of all ages and stages of their relationship. As young as John and Maria are, let's expand our lens and consider what may go on as they age and mature in themselves and in their relationship.

The next decade comprises crucial years, particularly for couples who come together as young people. John and Maria will continue to work on getting settled in their careers. They will have multiple opportunities to balance and support each other's climb up the ladder of achievement and success and the challenges that occur when this does not happen as expected. Again, there will be difficult decisions that have to be considered that can easily activate old unmet needs and longings.

Regarding having children, from the beginning of their relationship, they were both positive about wanting to have a family. While having a child is a joyful change, their differences in cultures and traditions will likely come into play and require new efforts and understandings. Even with a healthy child, the issues of a little one's biracial background will undoubtably be a factor that has to be understood. John will have to better understand his racial identity issues or else he may burden his child with these continuing internal conflicts. In addition, coming from very different family backgrounds, John and Maria will have to create ways of dealing with their families of origin. Such issues come to the foreground: How much do they see each of their families? How involved are they with their parents and other relatives? How much responsibility does this entail and how does the spouse feel about this? How does this affect their relationship as their parents age and possibly become impaired? Will John's feelings of pain and loss cause him to lapse into his obsession with porn again? Will Maria become punitive and rejecting, furthering John's need to withdraw into his efforts to soothe his pain alone?

When we bring ourselves to a relationship, our coping styles remain and are activated when we become frightened and feel unsafe. Given the attachment styles that we saw in Maria and John, we can assume that Maria will be the one to pursue and need John's involvement, while he may prefer to take refuge in work because it is less conflictual. Will they be able to remember what they learned in couples therapy? Will they continue to be curious about their raw spots when these arise and will they come together to fight their cycle of pulling apart? Based on the initial progress they made because of their commitment to their relationship, it seems hopeful that they will be able to create a deep enough connection that will help them stay and care, even when there are times of uncertainty and tension.

In the end, this book is about attachment and its enduring links that synchronize our heart to another person's heart. Poets and philosophers have written about this for as long as civilization exists.

In Conclusion

In our modern world we have attempted to examine and understand the components of this attachment that keep us connected but can cause us to come apart.

We have detailed the conversations and experiences of John and Maria with the hope that you can identify with their struggle whether you have had the same experience or not. We humans need to feel safe and secure if we are to be in a relationship with another human. John and Maria felt the biological pull of attraction but they had to find their way back into each other's heart by actually caring about what the other was going through. This process of deeply felt empathy is never automatic and it is not there every moment. It requires attention and interest sustained over time. As the relationship endures and is weathered by the passage of years, this commitment is a felt experience that acts as a buffer to the external challenges that all people face as aging occurs. What matters is that we know in our bones that as mammals we are sensitive, we are aware, and we feel the presence and attention from our partner. Without this presence and attention, like any living organism, we wither and stop functioning. John and Maria began the journey on this road of healing—of earning security. We are hopeful that they will continue to thrive and inspire you to do the same.

This book and the particular orientation that we have used to conceptualize the couple and our work as therapists is based on the experiences and knowledge that we have up to this point in time. Our understanding of human relationships, the human brain and our body is always expanding with new research and clinical knowledge. We hope that what we have suggested will remain relevant, but we know that there will be additional discoveries that will add to what we currently suggest. As humans our survival is based on being flexible and open to change. We want to emphasize this orientation to growth and enrichment of our knowledge as fundamental for all of us, as it was for John and Maria in building their relationship.

Questions for the Reader

The book is about the struggles of this couple. In reading about John and Maria's issues, are you able to identify issues you have in your partnership?

What feelings did you have as you learned and heard about John and Maria's conflict? Could you find yourself in their conflict?

Your feelings about conflict may be complex. Did your feelings change after you read about John and Maria?

How did you feel about John and why?

Can you imagine being John? How does that feel?

How did you feel about Maria and why?

Can you imagine being Maria? How does that feel?

If you have a partner, do you ever imagine how he/she feels?

What mistakes did you feel Maria made and what would you have done differently?

What mistakes did you feel John made and what would you have done differently?

How do you feel about their relationship and why? How quickly did you come to this conclusion and did it ever change?

How did you feel when John and Maria were in the midst of their repetitive dance? Do your feelings make sense to you in terms of your own lived experience?

John and Maria carried certain ways of relating. These ideas, not always conscious, were called internal working models and came from their early lived experiences. Can you identify your own internal working models that guide you in your relational experience?

Do you better understand couples therapy after learning about Maria and John's experience in couples therapy?

John and Maria were blindsided by their emotions. Does this ever happen to you and if so, what do you do when this happens?

John and Maria became more self-aware and vulnerable in the course of their therapy. They each became aware of their contribution to their conflict. If you reflect on your own process, what do you do well and what do you wish you did better?

Questions for the Reader

Our brain signals us when we are in danger, which is evident in Maria's angry reaction and John's pattern of withdrawal. When you think of yourself, what is your automatic tendency?

John talked about his bodily responses when he was having intense feelings. What do you know about your own body's response when you are having intense feelings?

John and Maria had difficulty communicating their feelings. How well do you believe you communicate your feelings? If you have a partner, what do you imagine he/she would say about this?

Maria was often very angry. What did you see Maria do, and how do you respond when you are angry?

How did John express fear, and how do you respond when you are afraid?

How did external forces (pandemic, immigration, employment, racial differences) affect John and Maria's relationship? Thinking of your own life, how do external forces affect your relationship?

Did you have any thoughts about the therapeutic process?
How did you feel about the therapist's personal thoughts and feelings?

How did you feel the therapist worked with John and Maria?

Do you have thoughts about what you feel the therapist could have done that would have been more helpful, more therapeutic, in working with John and Maria?

What are the main ideas from this book that you will remember and use?

REFERENCES

Beebe, B. and F. Lachman. (2002). Infant Research and Adult Attachment: Co-constructing interactions. Hillsdale, NJ: Analytic Press.

Bowlby, J. (1969). Attachment and Loss, Vol. 1: Attachment. New York: Basic Books.

Bowlby, J. (1979). The Making and Breaking of Affectional Bonds. London: Tavistock.

Brooks, D. (2011). The Social Animal: The Hidden Sources of Love, Character, and Achievement. New York: Penguin Press.

Cozolino, Louis. (2017). The Neuroscience of Psychotherapy: Healing the Social Brain, New York, W.W. Norton.

Goleman, D. (2005). Emotional Intelligence: Why It can Matter More Than I.Q. New York: Random House.

Gottman, J. and Nan Silver. (2015). The Seven Principles for Making Marriage Work. New York: Harmony.

Hazan C., and P.R. Shaver. (1987). Romantic Love conceptualized as an attachment process. Journal of Personality and Social Psychology 52: 511-24.

Jaffe, E. (2007). Mirror Neurons: How We Reflect on Behavior. Association for Psychological Science. May Issue.

Johnson, Susan. (2011). Hold Me Tight. London UK: Piatkus Books.

Lapides, Francine. (2011). The Implicit Realm in Couples Therapy: Improving Right Hemisphere Affect-Regulating Capabilities. Clinical Social Work Journal (2011) 39:161-169.

Lewis, T., Fari Amini and Richard Lannon. (2000). A General Theory of Love. New York: Vintage Books.

Main, Mary. (1995). Recent studies in attachment: overview with selected implications for clinical studies. In Attachment Theory: Social, Developmental, and Clinical Perspectives, ed. S. Goldberg, R. Muir, and J. Kerr. pp.407-474. Hillsdale, NJ: Analytic Press.

Marks-Tarlow, T. (Editor) (2020). A Fractal Epistemology for a Scientific Psychology. England: Cambridge Publishing.

Marks-Tarlow, T. (2015). The Nonlinear Dynamics of Clinical Intuition. Chaos and Complexity Letters 8: 1-24.

Siegel, D. J. (1999). *The developing mind.* New York, NY: Guilford Press

Schore, A. N. (2019). *The Development of the Unconscious Mind (Norton Series on Interpersonal Neurobiology).* New York: WW Norton.

Schroeder, M. (1991). Fractals, chaos, power laws: Minutes from an infinite paradise. New York, NY: W.H. Freeman & Company.

Solomon, M.F. (1994). Lean on Me: The Power of Positive Dependency in Intimate Relationships. New York: Simon & Schuster.

Taylor, S.E., L.C. Klein, et al.(2000). Biobehavioral responses to stress in females: Tend-and-befriend, not fight-or-flight. Psychol Rev 107(3): 411-29.

Tronick, E.Z. & Gianino, A. (1986). Interactive mismatch and repair: Challenges to the coping infant. Zero to Three, 6(3), 1-6.

About the Authors

Sondra Goldstein PhD is a clinical psychologist in private practice for over 40 years. Her doctoral study was at the University of Pittsburgh where she earned her PhD in 1971. She was a Clinical Associate Professor in the UCLA Department of Psychology from 1995-2017. For many years she was a member of Dr. Allan Schore's seminar focused on neuropsychology in psychotherapy. She currently studies with Dr. Terri Marks-Tarlow on the application of systems theory and creativity in psychotherapy. She has extensive training in Emotionally Focused Therapy and couples therapy, and enjoys seeing couples in her practice. Married for 52 years, her experience of living with her husband constantly creates appreciation and understanding of the challenges and rewards of a lasting couple relationship.

Susan Thau PhD, PsyD a licensed clinical psychologist and psychoanalyst, a wife, mother and grandmother, treats individuals, couples and families, working intensively with the emotional states of her clients. Dr. Thau believes that secure attachments and emotional self-awareness are the basis of feeling stable, secure and engaged in one's internal life and in relationships. Dr. Thau practices in Los Angeles and is part of an active and engaged therapeutic community that nourishes and sustains her therapeutic work.

Acknowledgments

This book has been a labor of love, coming out of our deep commitment to understand the inner world of the people we work with. Our journey to link our hearts and brains to the deep emotions that we all feel, has been fueled by many colleagues and supportive others in our community.

About twenty years ago, we began our work with Allan Schore PhD, participating in a study group focused on affect regulation and attachment. Allan's expertise and encouragement lead to our involvement in studying, speaking and writing about these theories and how they are most evident in couple relationships.

The genesis of this book was conversations with Donn Peters PsyD to make couples therapy more understandable to the lay public.

We began training with The International Center for Excellence in Emotionally Focused Therapy (EFT) founded by Susan Johnson EdD. We served on the first Board of Directors of the Los Angeles EFT Center working with James Furrow, PhD, who significantly deepened our understanding of attachment and emotional functioning and whose guidance has significantly influenced our work.

We also acknowledge and recognize other colleagues who have been an important part of our learning process: Nancy Gardner PhD, Karen Shore, PhD, Robert Ogner LCSW, Veronica Thomas PhD , James McCracken DCSW, and Rachel Thomas LMFT. Ongoing online training, the EFT Café, under the direction of Kathryn Rheem EdD, LMFT and Jennifer Olden MFT has informed our work. Jennifer's encouragement helped bring this book to fruition.

Ellen Neuborne, a writer and editor, extended expert advice and direction that helped this publication come to life. Ellen directed us to the Jenkins Group where Leah Nicholson, Yvonne Roehler, and Emily Slater brought our ideas into print and Kindle form.

We also want to thank a group of wonderful supporters who read and discussed the concepts for our book: Linda Lucks, Orlando Nava and Damion Dormeyer. Their comments and questions were invaluable in helping us focus and clarify the direction we had chosen.

We are grateful for the encouragement and endorsement of the value of this writing by Nancy Gardner PhD, Jeff Katzman MD, Jennifer Olden MFT, and Terry Marks-Tarlow PhD.

For us this book could not have come to completion without the understanding, patience and continuous encouragement of our husbands, Earl Goldstein and Bob Thau. Their steadfastness helped us persevere.

Lastly, we are grateful to the many couples and individuals we have worked with over the years who have taught us so much about the rollercoaster of emotions in relationships

Now we turn to you, our readers, and hope that you will be inspired to delve deeper into your own internal world that truly makes you who you are.

With immense thanks to all who made this book possible,

Sondra Goldstein and Susan Thau